Devotions for Dieters

A 365 Day Guide
To A Lighter You!

Dan R. Dick

Barbour and Company, Inc.
164 Mill Street
Westwood, New Jersey

OTHER Books by Dan R. Dick

WISDOM FROM THE BIBLE - Daily Thoughts
From the Proverbs

DAILY PRAISE FROM THE BIBLE - Inspiration
From the Psalms

DEDICATION:

To Lezlie,
who has proven
it can be done,
and
To Nancy,
who stands beside me
through thick and thin.

Contents

January: Holiness 1

February: Temptation 15

March: Courage 27

April: Patience 41

May: Faith 53

June: Hope 67

July: Perseverance 81

August: Comfort 95

September: Doubt 107

October: Strength 119

November: Joy and Thanksgiving 133

December: Victory 145

JANUARY

Holiness

We are created in God's image. He has given us a precious gift: the gift of life. When we truly appreciate that gift, we are compelled to do everything in our power to protect and preserve it. When we allow our bodies to get soft and unfit, then we are saying to God that His gift really doesn't mean anything to us. Poor physical condition that is due to our own negligence or laziness is an insult to our Creator. John the disciple claims that each of us is to strive to be perfect, as our Father in heaven is perfect. That perfection includes body and mind, not just spirit. To care for ourselves physically is to honor God and acknowledge our gratitude to God for the gift of life. Holiness can only come through discipline and obedience. Dieting requires both. We can learn to train ourselves as disciples through our bodily sacrifices. To care for our appearance and health is pleasing to God, and He will bless us richly in our endeavors.

January 1

"What? know ye not that your body is the temple of the Holy Ghost which is in you, which ye have of God, and ye are not your own? (1 Corinthians 6:19.)

As Christians, we believe that God dwells within us. Our bodies become His home, and it makes sense that we should try to make His surroundings as nice as possible. The temple of God in Israel was kept immaculately clean and pure. Only the most clean and holy of men were allowed to enter it. It was revered by all. The temple was the most holy and special place of all. When we are told that our bodies are the temple of God, it is not an option whether or not we will take care of it; it is a duty. When we care for our physical being, we are making God's temple a holy and special place.

Today's thought: We diet not only for ourselves, but for God!

January 2

. . . it is written, Be ye holy; for I am holy (1 Peter 1:16).

Too often we think that holiness is merely a matter of the spirit. We feel that if we read our Bible, pray regularly, and attend worship, we are being holy. But holiness requires that we tend to our physical health as well as our spiritual health. Early Christians realized that they were more alert and better able to concentrate on God when they felt good. Tending to the body made them better at their spiritual pursuits. Dieting may make us look better, but it will also make us feel better, and it will enable us to pursue God in deeper and more meaningful ways.

Today's thought: We please God when we try to be the best we can be!

January 3

For God hath not called us unto uncleanness, but unto holiness (1 Thessalonians 4:7).

When we try to figure out what it means to be holy, we think of many things that we do which we shouldn't. Our minds fill with "thou shalt nots" and we promise ourselves that we will do better. Our minds should not be so filled by the bad things we have done; we should focus on the good things we can do. Certainly, dieting requires sacrifice, but the benefits involved far outweigh the costs. Our focus must be on what we receive rather than what we must do without. Dieting is not turning from what we shouldn't do. Dieting is doing what God calls us to do.

Today's thought: God will not leave us when we respond to His call!

January 4

For ye are bought with a price: therefore glorify God in your body, and in your spirit, which are God's (1 Corinthians 6:20).

Sometimes it is difficult to stick with a diet once it has begun. If we are dieting for ourselves, we often lose heart, but if we feel we're dieting for someone else, it can be the motivation we need to stick with it. Everyday we make promises to God, and those promises we do everything in our power to keep. God calls us to be the best we can be, physically as well as spiritually. We should commit our diets to God. If we see dieting as a sacrifice we make to God, then we can find a deeper power to remain committed to our efforts to lose weight. Let everything we do honor and glorify God, for that is what truly pleases him.

Today's thought: We are not alone in our attempt to lose weight!

January 5
If we confess our sins, he is faithful and just to forgive us our sins, and to cleanse us from all unrighteousness (1 John 1:9).

Once we decide for ourselves that being overweight is wrong, then it is vital that we put ourselves in God's hands. Though being overweight is not a sin, few people would say it is good. We should avoid everything that is not good. God will help us whenever we turn from things that are bad. Prayer is an important part of our attempts to lose weight. We can trust God to bless all our efforts to do what we feel is right. There is no reason to feel guilty for being overweight, for God forgives us our weakness and offers His own strength as our own. We can start our diets with a clear conscience and an assurance that God is with us every step of the way.

Today's thought: We have nothing to feel guilty about!

January 6
And almost all things are by the law purged with blood; and without shedding of blood is no remission (Hebrews 9:22).

If we learn anything at all from being a Christian, we learn that good things do not come without sacrifice. Jesus had to give everything He had in order to reunite us with God. If we decide to be the best we can be, then we need to accept the fact that there is some sacrifice required. When we learn to sacrifice, we learn what it means to be Christian. Sacrifice is a good discipline. Sacrifice teaches us what is really important, and it helps us be thankful for what we have. When we stop to think of how great Christ's sacrifice for us was, it inspires us in our diets to become better people; people worth dying for!

Today's thought: Dieting can draw me closer to being a disciple!

January 7
But now in Christ Jesus ye who sometimes were far off are made nigh by the blood of Christ (Ephesians 2:13).

A friend of mine who was dangerously overweight lamented to me once that she was "so fat that God wouldn't even recognize me as the person He created." She felt that her weight problems had driven a wedge between her and God. How sad. Nothing that we do ever really separates us from God, but when we feel badly about ourselves, we feel we are unlovable, even by God. It is important that we see ourselves as good people. God loves us no matter how we look, but He is delighted with us when we take pride in who He created us to be. God will bless our efforts, so we need to draw as close to Him as possible as we attempt to diet.

Today's thought: God loves us just as we are.

January 8

This is that bread which came down from heaven: not as your fathers did eat manna, and are dead: he that eateth of this bread shall live for ever (John 6:58).

Face it: Dieting wouldn't be so hard if food didn't taste so good! Like anything good, we want to get as much of it as we can. It's easy to place a high value on the food we eat. But, there is such a thing as too much of a good thing. God has given us many freedoms, but one we should not abuse is the freedom to consume as much food as we want. No one can limit what we eat except ourselves. We need to realize that our daily bread supplies what we need, not what we want. Excessive eating is selfishness, and selfishness is sin. When we feel the urge to overeat, let us turn to God and nourish ourselves on the true bread that comes from Him — His word.

Today's thought: God's bread of life is nonfattening!

January 9

For bodily exercise profiteth little: but godliness is profitable unto all things, having promise of the life that now is, and of that which is to come (1 Timothy 4:8).

There is an old adage that says, "Don't put the cart before the horse." Many people try to lose weight without a specific goal in mind. Often people set a goal that is unrealistic. In our attempts to become more Christian, we grow a little at a time. God doesn't expect us to be perfect right away. He knows that our growth takes time. The same is true of our attempts to lose weight. We need to take it a little at a time. Crash diets and heavy exercise programs are not the way to go. Our Christian growth should provide us with an example. Let us approach our diets with patience and take it a small step at a time.

Today's thought: Dieting is easier if we try to lose weight little by little.

January 10

And be not conformed to this world: but be ye transformed by the renewing of your mind, that ye may prove what is that good, and acceptable, and perfect, will of God (Romans 12:2).

The stomach is a spoiled brat. When we miss even one meal, it kicks up a fuss and makes us feel as though we're going to starve. Of course, we're in no danger whatsoever, but once our stomachs get started, it is hard to ignore them. To diet means to engage in mind over matter. We need to realize that we can get by on a lot less food than we actually eat. We need to renew our mind, change our thinking, and decide that we're not going to be made a slave to our stomachs. We resent it when someone else tries to control us. Why should we so easily succumb to our own stomachs? When we refuse to be ruled by anything but the Spirit of God, then we truly please Him.

Today's thought: God can liberate us from slavery to the stomach!

January 11

And the peace of God, which passeth all understanding, shall keep your hearts and minds through Christ Jesus (Philippians 4:7).

When I get hungry, I get nervous and anxious. I find that I snap at people and have a very short temper. This is an indication that food is more than just a pleasure; it is an addiction. To kick an addiction requires restraint and peace. Jesus Christ promises blessed peace and rest to all who come to Him. It is important for us to rely on the gentle comfort of God when we face the trials of dieting. God knows what we are going through, and He rejoices when we turn to Him for peace of mind and heart. It is not vital that we understand how this peace can come to us. What is important is that we truly believe God will grant it.

Today's thought: In God, there is peace that is greater than the turmoil caused by our dieting!

January 12

Draw nigh to God, and he will draw nigh to you. Cleanse your hands, ye sinners; and purify your hearts, ye double minded (James 4:8).

Dieting involves a constant struggle between two intense desires: the desire to lose weight and the desire to indulge in the foods we love. This is not an easy struggle. We are doubleminded. God wants all of His children to learn to be singleminded. Once we decide that something is important, we should learn to stick to it. That's not easy to do on our own. For that reason, it is helpful for us to draw close to God. He will listen as we tell our troubles. The closer we are to God, the more He can help us through difficult times. If we ask Him to, God will help us become singleminded. He is as anxious as we are to see us attain our goal.

Today's thought: God will keep us on the right track!

January 13

He that followeth after righteousness and mercy findeth life, righteousness, and honour (Proverbs 21:21).

Long-distance runners train themselves to think of the finish line. They visualize it just ahead. They say this keeps them from wanting to give up somewhere along the way. The reward of crossing the finish line is worth more than any pain or discomfort on the way. Dieters can learn from this. Instead of dwelling on how hungry we are, or how much we long for rich foods, we should continually think in terms of the rewards that await us at the end. Christians follow Christ with hope of a heavenly reward. Faith means we await something yet to come. Dieting means we live in the hope of trimming down and looking fit.

Today's thought: The reward of our diet is greater than the sacrifice!

January 14

For the righteous Lord loveth righteousness; his countenance doth behold the upright (Psalms 11:7).

Don't let self-pity become part of your diet. It's very easy to feel sorry for yourself when you diet. First, you feel bad because you're overweight. Then you feel bad because of all you have to give up. You feel badly because other people don't seem to understand what you're going through. They get to eat as they please. All of these things can make dieters feel extremely sorry for themselves. Take heart. God knows what you're going through, and He is delighted that you care so much about yourself. It is right and good to want to lose weight. Whenever we try to do what we think is right, God supports us completely. Replace self-pity with the blessed assurance that God is on your side.

Today's thought: Dieting is no reason for self-pity!

January 15

For the eyes of the Lord run to and fro throughout the whole earth, to shew himself strong in the behalf of them whose heart is perfect toward him. Herein thou hast done foolishly: therefore from henceforth thou shalt have wars (2 Chronicles 16:9).

My grandfather always said to me, "You plant your field, you have to harvest it." We made ourselves overweight, and we either have to live with it or work to change it. It is foolishness to over-indulge, but that doesn't stop us from doing it. Anyone who is overweight knows well that we have to pay for our foolishness. True wisdom comes from God. When we decide that enough is enough, that it is time to lose weight, we can know God will help us, especially through the toughest times. All we need do is ask. God is looking for ways to help us, but He always waits until His help is invited. Don't hesitate. Call upon the Lord, and He will hear you.

Today's thought: If we turn from our foolishness, God will bless us!

January 16

I am come a light into the world, that whosoever believeth on me should not abide in darkness (John 12:46).

When we feel bad about ourselves, we tend to dwell under a dark cloud of depression. Sometimes we can't think of anything else but how much weight we've gained and how much we would like to lose. The good news is that darkness always is replaced by light. We can get out from under the burden of our weight. We can change for the better. Our Lord is a liberator. He frees us from anything that oppresses us. Obesity is oppressing, and God is ready and willing to free us. No darkness is too great for God to dispel. No matter how dark and dismal our physical condition may be, in the light of Christ, we can trim down.

Today's thought: We always look better in God's light than in our own darkness.

January 17

The Lord knoweth the days of the upright: and their inheritance shall be for ever (Psalms 37:18).

God honestly does know what we suffer through when we try to lose weight. He sympathizes with us in all our suffering, but He can also see the prize that awaits us. He knows the inheritance that is to come. Even when we have difficulty keeping our eyes focused on the goal, we can turn to God, who will strengthen us by His own strength. He always sees us as what we can potentially be: slim, trim, and healthy. It is important for us to try to see ourselves the same way God sees us. Remember, once weight is lost, the struggle is not completely over, but we need not ever return to obesity. The fruits of our labors, our inheritance, can last forever.

Today's thought: God wants to see us achieve our goal!

January 18

. . . Be it far from me; for them that honour me I will honour, and they that despise me shall be lightly esteemed (1 Samuel 2:30).

A friend of mine played basketball in high school. He did everything he could to become the best player he could be. He worked with the coach every day. He respected the coach and did everything the coach told him, in order to please him. His hard work paid off. He starred on the team, and when he graduated, the coach told him he was the finest player he had ever had the privilege of coaching. Are we doing everything we can to please God by being the best people we can be? When we diet, we do God honor, and He will be faithful to honor us in return. If we ignore our bodies, the gift that God gave us, then we show contempt for God, and He will lose respect for us.

Today's thought: Today I will do everything I can to please God!

January 19

. . . because Christ also suffered for us, leaving us an example, that ye should follow his steps . . . Who his own self bare our sins in his own body on the tree, that we, being dead to sins, should live unto righteousness . . . (1 Peter 2:21, 24).

It is good for us to remember, as we sit feeling sorry for ourselves because we may not indulge in tasty pleasures, that our sacrifice is not really so great when we compare it to the many sacrifices Christ made. What we are doing is indeed a sacrifice, but for self rather than for others. Christ sacrificed for us in order that we might enjoy life to the fullest. Let us learn from the sacrifice of Christ and remember that He has given us the power to overcome any temptation that might present itself.

Today's thought: Christ has conquered temptation and will be with me!

January 20

. . . if thou shalt confess with thy mouth the Lord Jesus, and shalt believe in thine heart that God hath raised him from the dead, thou shalt be saved (Romans 10:9).

Talk to Jesus. Seriously, He is waiting to listen to you and help you in your struggle to lose weight. Sometimes we wrestle with the urge to cheat on our diets until we are emotional wrecks. This happens most often when we are alone, with no one to talk to. Don't forget, Christ is always with you, and He is as close as a prayer. Tell Him how difficult it is. Let Him know your struggle, and He will indeed comfort you. There is never a time in our lives when Jesus is not interested in everything that is happening to us. Call upon Him, confess Him as Lord, and you will be saved!

Today's thought: Jesus is as close as a prayer!

January 21

. . . but ye are washed, but ye are sanctified, but ye are justified in the name of the Lord Jesus, and by the Spirit of our God (1 Corinthians 6:11).

In many respects, dieting is like a washing away of fat. What greater joy is there than to step up on the scales and see the pointer a few marks to the left of where it was a couple days before. When we lose, we feel cleansed, and the cleansing is not just physical. Emotionally we begin to feel better about ourselves. Our guilt, our poor self-image, our pain all begin to wash away, too. This is the best washing of all. We are renewed both inside and out, and we become a fitting and holy temple; a righteous dwelling place for the Lord!

Today's thought: Each pound lost cleanses me physically, spiritually, and mentally.

January 22

Therefore if any man be in Christ, he is a new creature: old things are passed away; behold, all things are become new (2 Corinthians 5:17).

Some people say that what we look like on the outside has nothing to do with what we're like on the inside. This is true to a degree, but how we see ourselves has very much to do with what we think of ourselves. If we see ourselves as overweight, we will tend to think less of ourselves. If we see ourselves as physically fit and trim, then we will feel better. One of the advantages of leaning on Christ when we diet is that He has the power to make the old pass away and to bring about a wonderful newness to our lives. No one wants our transformation more than Christ Jesus. He's there to help.

Today's thought: There's a brand new me on the way!

January 23

The Lord rewarded me according to my righteousness: according to the cleanness of my hands hath he recompensed me (2 Samuel 22:21).

Don't expect God to make you thin. You have to do the hard part for yourself. Do know this, however: God will bless you beyond your wildest hopes if you will put forth your best effort and not give up. When we show Him that we really are serious about being better people, He is pleased beyond measure, and He will do all kinds of wonderful things to help us along. When we refuse to give into the temptations, to dirty our hands, then God will reward us and lift us up. All He asks is that we give it our very best effort. If we do that, we will succeed.

Today's thought: God is pleased by my best effort to lose weight.

January 24

Righteousness shall go before him; and shall set us in the way of his steps (Psalms 85:13).

Jesus fasted forty days in the wilderness, and He was sustained by His faith. The devil came to Him and tried to tempt Him with bread, but He refused to give in. This is a good image for us to remember when we are dieting. Often we feel we cannot go on when we miss just one meal. Christ proved to us that even after missing meals for forty days, there is still a source of strength other than food. That source is God, and His strength is available to everyone who will ask for it. Let us remember to follow in the steps of Jesus Christ and lean on our heavenly Father whenever we feel weak or tempted.

Today's thought: I am facing nothing that Christ did not face before me.

January 25

Commit thy works unto the Lord, and thy thoughs should be established (Proverbs 16:3).

A woman I know carried a pocket New Testament with her wherever she went. Often I would see her pull it out of her pocketbook and begin reading. One day I asked her why she seemed so intent on her reading whenever I saw her. She said, "I read it whenever I get hungry. I'm trying to control my weight, so whenever I feel a physical hunger, I feed myself spiritually instead. It takes my mind off my hunger and puts it where it should be — on the Lord." What a wonderful lesson. If we will find new ways to include God in our diet, He will turn our thoughts where they need to be!

Today's thought: There are ways to be fed (spiritually) without getting fat!

January 26

Blessed are the pure in heart: for they shall see God (Matthew 5:8).

Once we decide something is wrong, (being overweight, for example), then doing that thing is sinful. Some may say, "Well, the Bible doesn't say obesity is a sin." The Bible does tell us that anything we do that makes us less than God created us to be is a sin. To be pure in heart means to try to do everything we know we ought to do. We ought to regard our own bodies with respect. We ought to be an example for others to follow. We ought to do all we can to be all we can. When we stay true to what we know in our hearts is right, then we will be assured of a place with God in His kingdom.

Today's thought: I will do all I can to be all I am meant to be!

January 27

For to be carnally minded is death; but to be spiritually minded is life and peace (Romans 8:6).

There is a gruesome children's story about a little girl who ate so much that she could no longer move. Then it began to rain, and she died of drowning. Sometimes we try to use terror tactics to get children to do what they should do and avoid things that are bad for them. By the time we're adults, we have forgotten the lessons we were taught as children. There is nothing of any lasting good to be gained from overeating. We need to turn away from what we know is bad, to something better. We need to take seriously the consequences of gluttony, and turn toward God, who will help us change our ways.

Today's thought: I must set my mind on more important things than food!

January 28

He shall send from heaven, and save me from the reproach of him that would swallow me up. God shall send forth his mercy and his truth (Psalms 57:3).

There are going to be days when we feel we just can't do it. Everywhere we turn, there is another temptation, another chance to blow it. Occasionally, we might even give in, but that's no reason to give up. Part of being human means we won't succeed every time we try something. That's okay. When we find ourselves in situations where we give in, that is when we need to call on God, asking for forgiveness, strength, and determination. God shall send forth His mercy and His truth, and we will be able to pick up from where we left off and do even better the next time.

Today's thought: Losing one battle doesn't mean I've lost the war!

January 29

If iniquity be in thine hand, put it far away, and let not wicked-ness dwell in thy tabernacles. For then shalt thou lift up thy face without spot; yea, thou shalt be stedfast, and shalt not fear (Job 11:14, 15).

A vegetarian friend of mine went to a party and was handed a plate filled with wonderful appetizers. He selected one, took a bite, and then — to everyone's surprise — he threw the remainder across the room with all his might. He stood with a stunned and bewildered look on his face. The appetizer had been filled with meat, and his immediate reaction was to throw it as far away as possible. I think of that whenever I am tempted to grab something to eat that I shouldn't have. In my mind, I have to throw it far away, acting like it is something terrible, so I won't give into the temptation.

Today's thought: I will put far away anything that tempts me this day!

January 30

God is our refuge and strength, a very present help in trouble (Psalms 46:1).

My grandmother had a favorite picture that showed Jesus stretching out His hand to Peter while they were walking on the sea. It gave my grandmother great comfort to know that if she ever failed in her faith, Christ would stretch out His loving hand to lift her up. Whenever she dieted, she kept that picture close at hand. When the diet got too hard for her to cope with, she looked at her picture and felt God present with her. When we attempt to sacrifice anything, it is good for us to admit that we will have a hard time doing it on our own. When we stretch forth our hand to God, He will always reach back.

Today's thought: When my diet gets toughest, God will be closest.

January 31

The wicked worketh a deceitful work: but to him that soweth righteousness shall be a sure reward (Proverbs 11:18).

It seems too easy to cheat on a diet. There are so many good things to eat, and it doesn't seem like it could hurt to cheat just a little. The problem is, when we try to convince ourselves that a little cheating is okay, then we never seem to draw the line, and a little cheating becomes a lot of cheating. When we are deceitful with ourselves, we find ourselves in big trouble. It is much better for us to do what we know is right, avoiding the things we know will give us trouble. When we stick to our diets, then we can expect nothing but reward.

Today's thought: There's no such thing as cheating just a little!

FEBRUARY
Temptation

There are so many wonderful things to indulge in. No matter where we look, there are temptations abounding. The harder we try to resist temptation, the greater the temptation seems. When we diet, everything reminds us of food. Everywhere we turn, there are pictures, signs, advertisements, smells, sounds, and other reminders of what we are trying to give up. If we are honest, we will admit that we need help. God can be that help, if we will let Him. Jesus Christ faced amazing temptations in the wilderness. Satan faced Him directly, though he went away defeated. The same power that Jesus drew on is available to us. We, too, can defeat the temptations we come up against. Dieting is easier when we feel that we are not alone. Make dieting a partnership effort. Include God in your attempt to lose weight, and he will bless you with strength to withstand all temptation.

February 1

My little children, these things write I unto you, that ye sin not. And if any man sin, we have an advocate with the Father, Jesus Christ the righteous (1 John 2:1).

"I can't win," the woman lamented. "I give in and eat something, and then I feel guilty. When I feel guilty, I eat. The more I eat, the guiltier I feel, and the guiltier I feel, the more I eat!"

Sometimes we feel like failures when we break our diets. We can be swept up in a sense of guilt that makes it nearly impossible for us to stick to our diet. The solution to guilt is forgiveness, and forgiveness comes to us through our advocate, Jesus Christ the righteous. Jesus knows that we sometimes give in, and He loves us just the same. Accept His love, accept His forgiveness, and let go of any guilt you may feel.

Today's thought: I am not condemned just because I sometimes slip!

15

February 2

And by him all that believe are justified from all things, from which ye could not be justified by the law of Moses (Acts 13:39).

I knew a man who tried a new diet about every two months or so. He would buy the newest diet book and throw himself into the program wholeheartedly. For a week or so, he would remain faithful, then, when results didn't occur fast enough to suit him, he'd fall away. He would curse the diet plans, saying they were no good, completely ignoring his own responsibility to stick to the plan. A book, a law, or a set of rules won't have any effectiveness unless we remain faithful to it. The desire to succeed won't come from a book; it needs to come from a deeper source. For us, that source is Jesus Christ.

Today's thought: Christ is better than any diet book!

February 3

Now unto him that is able to keep you from falling, and to present you faultless before the presence of his glory with exceeding joy (Jude 24).

There was a girl by the name of Jennifer who was always getting herself into trouble because she couldn't say no. She had absolutely no resistance to any temptation. Then she met Beth. Beth was able to be a voice of reason and common sense for Jennifer. Jennifer knew that if she was tempted, Beth would get her through. Jesus Christ can be to us what Beth was to Jennifer; He can be our voice of reason. Whenever we feel ourselves being tempted, we need to turn toward Him. He is able to keep us from falling. When we find ourselves too weak to handle a situation, we can rest assured that Jesus is indeed strong enough.

Today's thought: Jesus can keep me on the right track!

February 4

Iniquities prevail against me: as for our transgressions, thou shalt purge them away (Psalms 65:3).

I remember trying to fly a kite at the beach once. I would run as hard as I could in the sand, and it felt like I wasn't getting anywhere. I couldn't run fast enough to keep the kite aloft. Often dieting feels the same way. The harder we try, the farther we seem from our goal. It really doesn't seem worth all the effort it takes.

However, we need to hold on. When I tried to fly my kite, a sudden gust of wind came and took it high into the sky. The Holy Spirit of God comes to us just like a gust of wind, helping us reach our goals and making the result well worth the effort.

Today's thought: Jesus will give us the extra we need to lose weight!

February 5
Let the wicked forsake his way, and the unrighteous man his thoughts: and let him return unto the Lord, and he will have mercy upon him; and to our God, for he will abundantly pardon (Isaiah 55:7).

He loved fried food: meats, vegetables, fish — anything and everything fried. Now he was stuck. He promised his wife that he wouldn't eat any more fried food, but everytime he went into a restaurant, the old smells came to him and made both his mouth and eyes water. Time after time, he gave in and indulged in fried delights. Guiltily, he would admit his transgressions to his wife, who would scold him, forgive him, and force him to promise not to fall to the temptation again. Forgiveness is important for us to feel when we fall, but we shouldn't take advantage of it. We must always try our best to keep our promises and not ask forgiveness lightly.

Today's thought: We need fear no condemnation from God when we fall!

February 6
There hath no temptation taken you but such as is common to man: but God is faithful, who will not suffer you to be tempted above that ye are able; but will with the temptation also make a way to escape, that ye may be able to bear it (1 Corinthians 10:13).

There are going to be times when we feel like throwing up our hands and saying, "I just can't do it!" Dieting is not easy. Don't let anyone tell you that it is. We wouldn't need to diet if we could eat what we wanted when we wanted it. But know this: God will make sure we can hang on, if we include him in our diet attempts. He knows how hard it is and how much we struggle. No matter how tempted we might be, He will help us escape it.

Today's thought: There is a way to beat every temptation!

February 7

But I have prayed for thee, that thy faith fail not: and when thou art converted, strengthen thy brethren (Luke 22:32).

Everyone always wanted Brad on their team. He was tall and very athletic, and every team he ever played for seemed to win. There was also something about Brad that brought out the best in everyone else.

It's good to have someone on our side who can swing the odds in our favor. Jesus Christ is just that someone. He promised His disciples that He would pray for them and they could not fail in their endeavors. He prays for us, too. Jesus is always on our side, and that makes us unbeatable. As we attempt to lose weight, it is vital that we include Jesus in our plans.

Today's thought: With Jesus on my side, temptation doesn't stand a chance!

February 8

Submit yourselves therefore to God. Resist the devil, and he will flee from you (James 4:7).

The earliest days of a diet are the hardest. There are times when it just seems impossible to resist the wonderful treats that appear everywhere. But resist we must. The reward comes to us when we realize that with each victory over an individual temptation, it becomes all the easier to resist in the future. The largest part of the battle is to realize that we really *can* do it. The scriptures promise us that when we resist temptation (the devil), it will flee from us, and it will trouble us no more. God never makes a promise that He won't keep. The battle's been won.

Today's thought: There is no temptation I cannot resist!

February 9

For in that he himself hath suffered being tempted, he is able to succour them that are tempted (Hebrews 2:18).

When we get particularly low during our dieting times, we feel so alone and alienated. People pat us on the back and tell us they know how we feel, but we know they really don't. There are times we feel certain that no one knows how we feel. Rest assured, though, that Jesus knows how hard it is, and He wants to comfort us, especially when the going gets the toughest. Turn to Him, and

He will give you comfort and strength in the darkest times. He's been there before us, and He is willing to walk our path with us. Welcome Him in, and He will grant you comfort.

Today's thought: No matter how lonely I might feel, Jesus is right beside me!

February 10
He that overcometh shall inherit all things; and I will be his God, and he shall be my son (Revelation 21:7).

Being thin is a wonderful goal. Regaining health and vigor is also great. Looking and feeling good are important, but both pale in comparison with how good it is to please the Lord by being the best people we can be. When we diet, we not only gain physically, but also spiritually. Resisting temptation tones our spiritual being as well as dieting tones our physical being. When we reach our goal in our diet, we reach a second goal, as well: We do what is pleasing to God. When we are faithful to do the will of the Lord, we can rest assured that we have an eternal home with Him.

Today's thought: Dieting makes me a spiritual overcomer as well as a physical overcomer!

February 11
Be not overcome of evil, but overcome evil with good (Romans 12:21).

Fat is the enemy. We have declared war, and it takes every ounce of strength we have to wage the battle. Yet, it is a battle well worth fighting. We sometimes need to look at fat as an enemy. We need to think of it as evil, in order to stay serious about battling it. If we allow ourselves to believe that it is anything less than evil, we stand in danger of learning to live with it. That can never be. It is an affrontery to the Christian life to allow evil to overcome that which is good. Rather, let us always strive to overcome what is evil with what is good.

Today's thought: I will not rest until the enemy has been eradicated!

February 12
The Lord knoweth how to deliver the godly out of temptations, and to reserve the unjust unto the day of judgment to be punished (2 Peter 2:9).

I remember when I proposed to my wife, I wanted to call home and let everyone know. I called, but the line was busy. I was so excited that I just sat and kept dialing until I broke through. I must have called a hundred times before my efforts paid off. I finally got through because of persistence. Persistence is one of the most important ingredients of a successful diet. The Bible tells us often that God is pleased by our persistence, and He will reward us for it. God will deliver us, if we will keep trying no matter what happens. Just don't give up!

Today's thought: No matter what happens, I will keep trying to lose weight!

February 13

Blessed is the man that endureth temptation: for when he is tried, he shall receive the crown of life, which the Lord hath promised to them that love him (James 1:12).

What a great feeling! Kim had gone to the party dreading all the comments of her friends. When they found out she was on a diet, she knew her friends would try everything they could to get her to eat the scrumptious food that would be available. It hadn't been as bad as she thought it would be, though. Her friends had tried to tempt her, but she had resisted. It had been difficult, but now it felt great to know that she could be strong when she really needed to be. If she could resist the temptations of her friends, she could resist anything. For the first time since she started dieting, Kim began to really believe she could do it.

Today's thought: The Lord provides special strength for each new temptation!

February 14

There is therefore now no condemnation to them which are in Christ Jesus, who walk not after the flesh, but after the Spirit (Romans 8:1).

Perhaps the worst part of dieting is the guilt that accompanies the desire to break from the diet at any possible moment. For some, dieting becomes a challenge to see how sneaky a person can become, but inevitably guilt creeps in and spoils everything. Dieting requires a good spirit and a hopeful outlook. We cannot expect to maintain a good state of mind when we continually condemn ourselves for our failures. We need to resolve to try harder and then forget our failings. When we can forgive and forget, we stand a much better chance of a successful diet.

Today's thought: Valentine's candy adds to the flesh; the word of God is less fattening!

February 15

And he said unto me, My grace is sufficient for thee: for my strength is made perfect in weakness. Most gladly therefore will I rather glory in my infirmities, that the power of Christ may rest upon me (2 Corinthians 12:9).

The little boy tagged farther and farther behind his parents. As his father turned to tell him to hurry up, the little boy sobbed, "I can't hurry. I'm too tired. Carry me." He stopped where he was and lifted his weary little arms.

During our diets, we often feel just like that little boy. We just can't go on anymore; we just don't have the strength. That's when we need to turn to God. In our weakness he brings us strength. You will be amazed at what great endurance the Lord gives to those who stretch out their arms to Him.

Today's thought: The Lord lifts us up from temptation when we reach out to Him.

February 16

And thine ears shall hear a word behind thee, saying, This is the way, walk ye in it, when ye turn to the right hand, and when ye turn to the left (Isaiah 30:21).

Diet plans come and go. Weight comes off, weight goes back on. One thing will not change, and that is the lovingkindness of the Lord. When the frustration sets in, the Lord is there. When we lose our patience, He will offer us His comfort. When we weaken and give in, He will forgive. The Lord is our closest ally and our strongest supporter. We may decide that a particular diet plan isn't for us, or that we need to try something new, but we can never afford to turn away from God. God will help us with whatever plan we choose to follow.

Today's thought: Any attempt I make to lose weight is incomplete without God!

21

February 17

These things I have spoken unto you, that in me ye might have peace. In the world ye shall have tribulation: but be of good cheer; I have overcome the world (John 16:33).

Sometimes we just get tired of dieting. It takes a lot of energy to diet, and without the foods we love, we're sometimes too weak to fight any longer. Our diets become bigger and bigger burdens. If we're not careful, we can lose sight of the fact that our diet won't last forever. All things come to an end if we will only be patient enough to wait. It helps to remember the temptations of Christ; how He triumphed over them, and then, before long, how they ended. Dieting is not punishment, but discipline. Though it can be a tribulation, losing weight carries with it a special joy.

Today's thought: As the fat fades, so does the tribulation!

February 18

And the God of peace shall bruise Satan under your feet shortly (Romans 16:20).

I remember going to a cafeteria with my friend once while I was on a diet. I told my friend that I was only going along to keep him company, but that I wouldn't eat anything. Once there, however, I was drawn to a particular piece of German chocolate cake. I debated with myself for the longest time, then finally gave in and went to the counter to buy it. On my way back to my seat, I turned too quickly, and the cake fell from my tray to the floor, where I proceeded to step on it. I always felt that perhaps God was trying to teach me something. The source of my temptation did indeed end up under my feet!

Today's thought: Food wasted is better than food waisted!

February 19

To him that overcometh will I grant to sit with me in my throne, even as I also overcame, and am set down with my Father in his throne (Revelation 3:21).

The ultimate goal of our Christian walk is to be like Jesus. The ultimate goal of our diet is to be trimmer and more fit. Both goals require great discipline and commitment. Both goals carry valuable rewards with them. It makes sense to combine the goals whenever we can. If we will diet prayerfully, constantly relying on

Jesus Christ for comfort and strength, then we will please the Lord and lose weight at the same time. With Christ we become overcomers, and we are promised that we will share in Christ's reward in our heavenly home!

Today's thought: I cannot be beaten, as long as Christ is on my side!

February 20
Commit thy way unto the Lord; trust also in him; and he shall bring it to pass (Psalms 37:5).

Alice Layden was a woman with no self-control. As long as I knew her, she had been terribly overweight. I hadn't seen Alice for over two years when she showed up one day on my front doorstep. She looked fabulous! When I asked how she had finally done it, she said, "I asked God to help me, and I just kept asking Him. Every morning, every noon time, each evening, and anytime I felt hungry, which was almost all the time, I just said a little prayer for God to get me through. He did it! After I thought I'd just about run out of things to try, I found what I should have known all along. God did for me what I was unable to do for myself!"

Today's thought: The more time spent in prayer, the less time left to eat!

February 21
It was therefore necessary that the patterns of things in the heavens should be purified with these; but the heavenly things themselves with better sacrifices than these (Hebrews 9:23).

I took a youth group to a play on Good Friday once while I was fasting. All I could think of was how hungry I felt. I was a little cranky, and I found it difficult to concentrate on the play. Suddenly, I looked at the face of the young man who played Christ. His face was contorted with the pain and suffering of our Lord. I looked at a face which truly mirrored everything Jesus had been through, and I was ashamed at myself for the self-pity I had indulged in. When I compared my minor discomforts with the true sufferings of Jesus, I realized I had nothing whatsoever to complain about.

Today's thought: I will think of what I have, rather than what I have not!

February 22

Casting all your care upon him; for he careth for you (1 Peter 5:7).

David was driving everyone crazy. He seemed to breeze through his diet while everyone else struggled. At first, everyone assumed he was cheating on his diet, but when he began losing weight faster than everyone else, they gave up on that thought. It was finally discovered that only one thing made David different from the rest of the group: David was a Christian. He began sharing his faith and told the others they could cast all their cares on the Lord and God would help them face all their trials and temptations. The group not only lost weight, they gained faith!

Today's thought: As we cast our cares on God, He casts His love on us!

February 23

The name of the Lord is a strong tower: the righteous runneth into it, and is safe (Proverbs 18:10).

Kate was so thankful that Dennis was willing to spend time with her. Since whe started her diet, Kate had tried everything in her power to keep from being alone. When she was alone, she ate. When she was with friends, she didn't feel the need quite as strongly. When she was with friends who understood her, they helped her keep her mind off food. Dennis was one of those understanding friends. He would talk and laugh and make her forget all about eating. He made himself available as much as he could, and Kate was truly grateful. She felt he was a fortress she could run to, where she would be safe from the temptations of food and drink.

Today's thought: God gives us places of refuge when we tire!

February 24

Let no man say when he is tempted, I am tempted of God: for God cannot be tempted with evil, neither tempteth he any man (James 1:13).

A woman I knew once told me, "If God wants me thin, He'll make me thin. Besides, He wouldn't have made so many tempting things if He didn't want me to eat them." The poor woman took no personal responsibility for herself, and within a year of our conversation, she was dead. Her heart just couldn't take the strain any more.

Though God will be faithful to help us, He will not do it all Himself. He does not tempt us, nor does He cruelly tease us. He wants only to help us, but we must want to help ourselves.

Today's thought: God is not the source of temptation, just the solution!

February 25

A little that a righteous man hath is better than the riches of many wicked (Psalms 37:16).

"I know my limits," Jean said. "If I only keep a little food in the house, then I won't be tempted to eat too much. If I stock up, I just know I'll end up stuffing myself. It's better to just avoid the temptation altogether."

Often it is better to avoid our temptations rather than try to face them head-on. We cannot enter into gluttony if we restrict the amount of food we keep on hand. Often our diets are made successful because of the preventive measures we take.

Today's thought: Knowing our limits helps us limit our wants!

February 26

For whatsoever is born of God overcometh the world: and this is the victory that overcometh the world, even our faith (1 John 5:4).

The greatest enemy we face as we diet is not food, or the gnawing hunger we endure. No, the greatest enemy we face is the lack of faith we have in ourselves. When the going gets tough, our tendency is to throw up our hands in surrender. That cannot be allowed to happen. As faithful people, we are tied to a special power that comes from beyond us. We are recipients of the holy power of God. That same power raised Christ from the dead and enabled Him to overcome every temptation that this world could throw at Him. With that kind of power, how can we fail at anything we do?

Today's thought: To diet means to do it!

February 27

That ye might walk worthy of the Lord unto all pleasing, being fruitful in every good work, and increasing in the knowledge of God (Colossians 1:10).

Joining the army requires good physical condition and discipline. This is especially true of the army of the Lord. God gave us our bodies, our minds, and our souls. They are tied closely together, and each is to be taken care of as well as we are able. There is no excuse for flabbiness of body, mind, or spirit. It is important that we strive not only to do what is good for our bodies, but also to avoid anything that might be detrimental. As we avoid temptation, we strengthen our wills and make them over in the image of our Lord Jesus Christ's own will.

Today's thought: When I look my best, I look most like Christ!

February 28

Cast not away therefore your confidence, which hath great recompence of reward (Hebrews 10:35).

Jeff came out of the store carrying the large package and shaking his head. He really hadn't wanted to buy the radio, but the salesman wouldn't take no for an answer. He had really been persuasive. After a few feeble attempts to resist, Jeff had finally given in. He just wasn't good at fighting off aggressive people. He needed confidence.

We need to be confident that what we do is right. When we lack the confidence we need, we are easy prey for temptation. Confidence is an important part of dieting. When we stand firm on what we have decided to do, then we will succeed.

Today's thought: Nothing can sway me from my diet, if I don't want it to!

February 29

I will instruct thee and teach thee in the way which thou shalt go: I will guide thee with mine eye (Psalms 32:8).

My mother cut out all between-meal snacks whenever weight became a problem for my sisters or me. She kept careful watch on us, to make sure our weight didn't get out of control. I resented it when I was young, but I sure appreciate it now. How wonderful it was to know that someone was watching out for me, making sure I didn't give into fattening temptations. God will do that for us if we let Him. He will twinge our consciences when we do what we should not, and we need to see that as blessing rather than curse. By heeding the voice within, we can conquer temptation and lose weight.

Today's thought: God sees every fattening move I make!

MARCH
Courage

Courage is not simply a quality of bravery for those who face insurmountable dangers. Courage is the ability to face unpleasant situations of all kinds. To diet requires great courage. We face many enemies when we try to lose weight. We are plagued by temptations, guilt, doubt, impatience, worry, and a host of other concerns. Only a person with rare devotion and courage will stand strong against such foes. The Lord is the source of great strength and courage. If we will include God in our weight-loss programs, we will be amazed at the courage He instills in us. As we meet the challenges of our diets, we find that we are better able to move forward, and our courage increases steadily. It is important to remember that all things are possible with the help of the Almighty God. When we feel least able to go on, God will provide us with the energy and drive to succeed.

March 1

And not only so, but we glory in tribulations also: knowing that tribulation worketh patience (Romans 5:3).

The growl of his stomach sounded like a ferocious beast. He felt light-headed and nervous. He kept telling himself that he couldn't really be hungry; it was just his imagination. The gnawing hunger would not abate. Before long he just felt like crying. As much as he wanted to lose weight, he just couldn't face the beast that growled in his midsection. In disgust, he pushed away from his desk and headed out to eat.

A hard part of dieting is showing our stomach who is boss. When our stomachs rule, we lose. Turn to the Lord when weakness sets in. He will see us through.

Today's thought: I'm not letting my stomach push me around anymore!

March 2

And the Lord, he it is that doth go before thee; he will be with thee, he will not fail thee, neither forsake thee: fear not, neither be dismayed (Deuteronomy 31:8).

Sylvia was such a support. She really did know what the other women were going through. Not so long ago, Sylvia had weighed well over two hundred pounds. If anyone had earned the right to speak, it was Sylvia. Somehow it made it easier having someone around who was both sympathetic to the struggle and had been successful. Sylvia was indeed a blessing.

It does help to have others around who have been down the road we are walking. These people can be a great source of comfort and courage. Thank God that these examples exist for us to follow. The Lord will not fail us.

Today's thought: I have no fear of failure, for the Lord is with me!

March 3

. . . teaching them to observe all things whatsoever I have commanded you: and, lo, I am with you alway, even unto the end of the world. Amen (Matthew 28:20).

A friend of mine fasts regularly, and to my astonishment, he never complains or seems to be the least bit ruffled by the experience. For myself, I find that fasting changes my whole disposition. I asked him his secret once, and he said, "It's no secret, really. All I do is pretend that the empty feeling in my stomach is really the Holy Spirit moving around, making itself comfortable inside. That way, the gnawing isn't unpleasant, but it's quite comforting to think that God is so very close." I tried to follow my friend's advice, and it has worked wonders for me. Try it today.

Today's thought: I will let my hunger turn my mind to God!

March 4

And call upon me in the day of trouble: I will deliver thee, and thou shalt glorify me (Psalms 50:15).

Jim's watch alarm beeped as the clock struck four. It sounded every hour and every half-hour. I turned to him and asked him what he had set so many alarms for.

"I'm on a diet. Every time my watch goes off, I take a moment to say a prayer to God. It may sound crazy, but it has made this the easiest diet I've ever tried. It calms me down and gets my mind off food for awhile. I feel like I've got a partner, and you know, it's always easier to do something when you don't have to do it alone."

Today's thought: I can be brave during the tough times, because God is with me!

March 5

And this is the confidence that we have in him, that, if we ask anything according to his will, he heareth us (1 John 5:14).

"God just doesn't want me to lose weight!" said Stephanie. "Each time I try, I fail. If God really wants me to lose weight, He'd help me."

Many people feel just like Stephanie. They think God isn't helping them because they aren't successful in their diets. The problem is that they want God to take the weight from them. That simply isn't the way God works. Instead, we need to know that He will work through us to make us strong enough to face the challenges and trials that await us. We take heart in knowing that God will not let us down and He will work with us all the way.

Today's thought: God will grant me courage that will not run out!

March 6

But the Lord is faithful, who shall stablish you, and keep you from evil (2 Thessalonians 3:3).

All her life she had tried to kid herself and say she didn't really have a weight problem. To admit she was fat would have been to admit that she needed to change her habits. She wasn't ready for that. Then her closest and dearest friend had a heart attack. It really scared her and forced her to look at the truth. She was fat, and nothing could change that fact unless she did something about it. It took a lot of courage to face the truth, but it seemed like a lot less courage than facing a possible heart attack. With God's help, she knew she could face the truth and change for the better.

Today's thought: God makes me fit to fight fat!

March 7

Being confident of this very thing, that he which hath begun a good work in you will perform it until the day of Jesus Christ (Philippians 1:6).

Confidence. There are days when we feel we don't even know the meaning of the word. It is hard to stay confident when we feel so weak. It is important that we realize where confidence comes from. Our confidence comes from the Lord. It comes from nowhere else. All we need do is look at the example of our blessed Lord, and we will see that He alone gives the kind of strength necessary to meet every challenge. The things He overcame cause our dieting efforts to pale in comparison. If Christ is truly our Lord and Master, then we will have confidence enough to succeed.

Today's thought: I am sure to lose weight because of Christ in me!

March 8
And it shall come to pass, that before they call, I will answer; and while they are yet speaking, I will hear (Isaiah 65:24).

When we feel the weakest and most vulnerable, then is the time to turn to God. God knows what we are up against, even before we call upon Him. There is no one who cares more about how we feel and how we do than God does. He is our staunchest supporter. He also realizes how difficult it is to face our diets alone. He waits for us to call on Him, but He will not force Himself on us until we call. When we do call, He will act quickly to help us, since He already knows what it is we will be asking. Don't hesitate! Call on God when you need Him most.

Today's thought: I am never out from under God's watchful eye!

March 9
Though I walk in the midst of trouble, thou wilt revive me: thou shalt stretch forth thine hand against the wrath of mine enemies, and thy right hand shall save me (Psalms 138:7).

I went through a terrible time when I first started dieting. Every once in awhile, I would get light-headed and my knees would buckle. It was not only embarrassing, but a bit frightening. When I spoke to the doctor about it, he told me it was just my mind playing tricks on me. He said my stomach was "mad at me" for taking away its extra food. I didn't need as much food, but psychologically, I wanted it. I left the doctor and went out to my car to pray. Whenever I felt the light-headedness start to creep in, I asked the Lord to revive me, and He did!

Today's thought: God is all the pick-me-up I need!

March 10

But and if ye suffer for righteousness' sake, happy are ye: and be not afraid of their terror, neither be troubled (1 Peter 3:14).

If the example of Jesus teaches us anything, it should be that suffering is a noble and good thing when it leads to a better way. Our diets are definitely the source of suffering, but there is great blessing awaiting all who stick with them. God has promised special blessing to those who keep courage in the face of suffering and don't give in. Losing weight not only makes us look and feel better, but it draws us closer to God and His divine plan for us. Our suffering is not in vain. It is all to the glory of the Lord.

Today's thought: I will fear nothing, as long as Jesus is with me!

March 11

And, behold, I am with thee, and will keep thee in all places whither thou goest, and will bring thee again into this land; for I will not leave thee, until I have done that which I have spoken to thee of (Genesis 28:15).

When I was little, I just hated to be alone. I was afraid of being by myself. When my family got a dog, it made my fear go away. There was never a time when I was alone again. Just having some other presence with me made a huge difference. Now that I'm grown up, I still have a constant companion who will never leave me alone. That companion is God. No matter what I do, I know I am not alone in the endeavor. My diet is no exception. When I feel the most alone, I just rely on the support of the Lord, and He gives me strength beyond measure.

Today's thought: God helps us to be the best we can be!

March 12

. . . The Lord is with you, while ye be with him; and if ye seek him, he will be found of you; but if ye forsake him, he will forsake you (2 Chronicles 15:2).

In this day and age, promises are made easily and just as easily broken. We promise ourselves that we are going to lose weight, then we turn around and cheat at every possible chance. For this reason, we ought to include God in our diets. Whereas we might break promises that we make to ourselves, we stand a much better chance of keeping the promises we make to God. When we break promises to ourselves, we have no one to answer to, but when we break our promises to God, He expects us to explain. Promising God that we will lose weight makes dieting much easier.

Today's thought: I will lose weight for God's sake!

March 13

But whoso hearkeneth unto me shall dwell safely, and shall be quiet from fear of evil (Proverbs 1:33).

Jesus faced many terrible experiences in His lifetime. The Bible tells of many incidents where crowds of people sought to kill our Lord. Whenever the pressures got too great, Jesus withdrew and spent time in prayer. That is an important lesson for us to learn. There will be times when the pressures build up while we try to lose weight. When the pressures get too much for us to handle, we should turn to the Lord in prayer. He will comfort us, strengthen us, and give us the courage we need to face every new day.

Today's thought: Jesus will take my mind off my diet!

March 14

Fear thou not; for I am with thee: be not dismayed; for I am thy God: I will strengthen thee; yea, I will help thee; yea, I will uphold thee with the right hand of my righteousness (Isaiah 41:10).

Will the diet ever end? That question gets asked an awful lot. What starts out as a good idea soon becomes torture. Giving up seems to be such a good idea. It's at those times that we need the most strength. We need something to pull us through the really tough times. The love of God is just what we need. God will give us strength and courage and will help us fight off the temptation to quit. Call upon the Lord, and He will uphold you, He will strengthen you, He will stay with you, no matter how tough the diet gets.

Today's thought: If I can make it through the tough times, I can make it through anything!

March 15

Therefore we are always confident, knowing that, whilst we are at home in the body, we are absent from the Lord (2 Corinthians 5:6).

David had never been able to stick to a diet. He had tried a number of times, but nothing seemed to help him lose weight. Then he met Jennifer. She was cute, and friendly, and thin. David was suddenly more ashamed of the way he looked than he had ever been before. He began a new diet, and this one worked. David's whole personality changed. he gained a new confidence and strength of will.

What we struggle with at one point becomes easy when we receive the right incentive. With God as our incentive, we can do wonders. Without God, we are helpless. With God, we can do all things.

Today's thought: I will make sure to keep God close by all day!

March 16

For our heart shall rejoice in him, because we have trusted in his holy name (Psalms 33:21).

The Psalms are a wonderful example of what it means to put trust in the Lord. David shared both his trials and his triumphs with his God. In every situation, David turned to God for guidance and support. David was a spiritual giant because he recognized the source of all that he was and could ever hope to be. We can be like David. If we will turn to God for His strength and courage in the face of our trials, He will provide for our every need. When we diet, we can rejoice in the fact that God will honor and bless our trust in Him.

Today's thought: The diet I keep will bring me joy and fulfillment!

March 17

He found him in a desert land, and in the waste howling wilderness; he led him about; he instructed him, he kept him as the apple of his eye (Deuteronomy 32:10).

It is vital that we remember how pleasing it is to God when we choose to lose weight. No matter how we look or act, God loves us, but just like earthly parents, when we do our best and look our best, we are most pleasing. God is proud of us when we sacrifice and learn self-discipline. He watches our every move, our every struggle, and He loves us. He will be with us continually. Let us follow His teachings and do all in our power to make Him proud of us; not only in our diets, but in every undertaking.

Today's thought: I am the nonfattening apple of God's eye!

March 18

. . . I am not ashamed: for I know whom I have believed, and am persuaded that he is able to keep that which I have committed unto him against that day (2 Timothy 1:12).

"You can't lose weight. You've never stuck with anything in your whole life." Those words haunt me all the time — everytime I slip and eat something I know I shouldn't. I hate it when people think I'm too weak to succeed in my diet. I hate it even more when I prove them right. Still, being ashamed of failing at my diet is often good for me. If I am ashamed enough, then it helps me stick with it the next time. God has helped me a lot to conquer negative shame. I have committed my diet to Him, and He is true to help me keep on track.

Today's thought: I'll prove to all my skeptical friends that I am capable of losing weight.

March 19

What shall we then say to these things? If God be for us, who can be against us? (Romans 8:31.)

Let's not call it *our* diet; let's call it *God's* diet. No, that doesn't mean God has to lose the weight. It means that we diet because it's what God wants of us. If it's God's diet, then God will help make sure that it goes well. He will bless those who diet in His name. It may sound silly to diet for God, but, as Christians, we are called to do everything in His name. When we live our lives as an offering to God, then we let the whole world know who gives us our strength and courage. If God is for us, then nothing can stand against us.

Today's thought: Dieting for God is a joy and a comfort!

March 20

As for me, I will call upon God; and the Lord shall save me (Psalms 55:16).

We went around the circle, telling about the diet plans we had tried. Most of the people said they had no luck, no matter what they tried. I was the only one who had succeeded in losing a considerable amount of weight. Everyone looked expectantly toward me when my time came. I smiled shyly and said, "The only thing that I did differently from any of you was to pray. I didn't trust any of the diet plans I saw, so I turned to God, instead. You all can try what you want to, but as for me, I'm going to keep putting my faith in God. He's why I'm thin now."

Today's thought: All else fails; try God!

March 21

Let your conversation be without covetousness; and be content with such things as ye have: for he hath said, I will never leave thee, nor forsake thee (Hebrews 13:5).

"I hate Sheila," Karen said. "Ever since she lost weight, she's been impossible to be around. She thinks she's so special."

Unfortunately, Karen suffered from a common problem. Sheila hadn't changed. Karen just felt guilty whenever Sheila came around, because she wasn't able to lose weight like Sheila had. Instead of sharing in Sheila's victory, Karen fell victim to jealousy and a bad conscience. Karen needs to understand that Sheila's victory is not her defeat. God will work with each of us where we are. It takes a brave person to celebrate when others succeed where we have not.

Today's thought: I will rejoice at the example of others who have lost weight!

March 22

For the mountains shall depart, and the hills be removed; but my kindness shall not depart from thee, neither shall the covenant of my peace be removed, saith the Lord that hath mercy on thee (Isaiah 54:10).

There are times when we feel God has left us to struggle on our own. No matter how we pray, how we plead, it seems no help will come to us. The temptations mount, and our strength and willpower get weaker and weaker. This is where faith comes in. In those times we feel God is absent from us, we must believe that He is still there. God will never leave us, no matter how we may feel. He stays constant for His children. Nothing can move God from our hearts, and we need to know that. God will give us strength in time of need. He will not abandon us, ever.

Today's thought: I may lose weight, but I can't lose God.

March 23

What man is he that feareth the Lord? him shall he teach in the way that he shall choose (Psalms 25:12).

A group at the church decided to help one another lose weight. A friend of one of the members joined the weight-loss group, even though he wasn't a Christian. After four or five sessions, the young man left the group, saying, "I thought we would help each other not eat. I didn't know you planned to pray and study the Bible. That junk won't help anyone." As it turned out, the group was quite successful. The young man failed because he wouldn't entertain the idea that God could be any help. Those who believe in God trusted in Him, and they were rewarded.

Today's thought: God is my secret weapon for success!

March 24

Draw nigh to God, and he will draw nigh to you. Cleanse your hands, ye sinners; and purify your hearts, ye double minded (James 4:8).

The cake looked great. Jim waited as long as he could, then, when his wife left the room, he grabbed a small piece. Thinking he would stuff it quickly into his mouth before his wife returned, he turned quickly, the cake fell from his hand. He reacted instinctively and snatched the falling cake. As his wife reentered, he tried to hide his cake-covered hand, but to no avail. He was caught, and there was no way to deny it. We need to stick to our diets and keep our hands clean of the foods we know we should avoid. Draw close to God and away from food. It's the best way.

Today's thought: If you cheat, you lose everything but weight!

March 25

And he said, My presence shall go with thee, and I will give thee rest (Exodus 33:14).

The most effective diets are those with planned "cheating" in them. Just as the children of Israel set aside a day for fasting from their daily bread, Christian dieters should set aside a day to indulge in the foods they enjoy. This makes the dieter more thankful for the special treats, as well as making the diet much more tolerable. It gives us something to look forward to, and it erases guilt from the process. We all need rest, and we will find new strength and courage when we break our diet fasts occasionally.

Today's thought: Even dieters deserve a day off.

March 26

The eternal God is thy refuge, and underneath are the ever-lasting arms: and he shall thrust out the enemy from before thee: and shall say, Destroy them (Deuteronomy 33:27).

It's strange to think of food as "the enemy," but that's the best way to look at it if we want to be effective in our diets. Taking off the pounds is a battle. In every battle we need ammunition. As Christians, our ammunition comes from the Spirit of God that dwells within us all the time. God becomes our fortress; our refuge against the assaults of fattening foods. If we think we can fight the battle alone, we will find it doesn't take long before we tire. At those times we will wish we had someone to take over. Thank the Lord that God is there, and He never tires of fighting alongside His children.

Today's thought: Dieting makes losers winners!

March 27

For the Lord God is a sun and shield: the Lord will give grace and glory: no good thing will he withhold from them that walk uprightly (Psalms 84:11).

I can remember a time when I was on the verge of tears because I was so hungry. I had fasted for almost five straight days, and some friends of mine walked in eating cheeseburgers. The smell assaulted my nose, and the sight of the burgers caused my stomach to clutch and growl. I look back on that incident now and realize that I could not have made it, if it hadn't been for the Lord.

When I think of God as my shield, I think of all the times I feel like giving up because I'm too weak to fight. At those times I'm all the more thankful that I have God to rest upon.

Today's thought: When my stomach attacks, God will defend me!

March 28

If we suffer, we shall also reign with him: if we deny him, he also will deny us (2 Timothy 2:12).

Jesus Christ arose from the dead, glorified and renewed. Before He could ascend to this glory, He had to suffer many things. Much in this life requires sacrifice and suffering before we can attain it. Ask any dieter. The road to thinness is a rugged one. Before we can stand up trimmer and healthier, we must buck up and buckle down. There is very little that is pleasant about dieting, except the end result. Jesus Christ understands what it means to sacrifice better than we ever can. By our sufferings we draw closer to Christ. One day we will reign with Him.

Today's thought: The power of Christ lifts me above all suffering!

March 29

So that we may boldly say, The Lord is my helper, and I will not fear what man shall do unto me (Hebrews 13:6).

In a prison camp, the people were starved for long periods of time. One man seemed unaffected by the treatment he received. While others complained about how hungry they were, this one man stood by silently. Finally, he was asked why he seemed to be doing so well while the others all suffered so. He replied, "I will not let my captors get the better of me. No matter what they do, they will not wear me down. I am the Lord's, and no one else has any power over my life. Men may take away my food, but only God can truly sustain me."

Today's thought: The need for bread is all in the head!

March 30

And who is he that will harm you, if ye be followers of that which is good? (1 Peter 3:13.)

Watch out! There are a lot of people who would take advantage of us, just because we are vulnerable. When we decide to lose weight, we find ourselves weak and looking for easy answers. Unscrupulous doctors, slick marketing gimmicks, and shyster con artists make promises and products purely for profit. They feed on poor people who want nothing more than the easiest way to take off pounds. Thank goodness we have a source of strength to resist such come-ons. God will protect us from running off after gimmicks and tricks. He is the true answer and the only way to succeed in everything we do.

Today's thought: No human plan or gimmick comes close to God's plan!

March 31

For ye shall go out with joy, and be led forth with peace: the mountains and the hills shall break forth before you into singing, and all the trees of the field shall clap their hands (Isaiah 55:12).

Our God is a God with a plan for His creation. Everything was created for a reason. God created us in His image, and His plan for us is to live a full, joyful, creative existence. We can best do this by keeping ourselves fit and trim and healthy. God rejoices, as does all His creation, when we live up to the potential He created in each one of us. When we succeed in our dieting attempts, we take a step toward fulfilling our purpose in life, and we go forth in joy and peace which passes any earthly joy or peace. Praise the Lord.

Today's thought: Thank you, Lord, for bringing me this far!

APRIL
Patience

There is no such thing as a "quick" diet. It takes time to put weight on, and it takes even more time to remove it. Dieting requires a great deal of patience, and patience is a virtue that too few people possess. When our patience begins to wear thin, we need to remember that God is only too willing to grant us a special measure of the divine patience He so sorely needs to deal with His people. Time passes slowly for people who diet. At times, it feels as though the clock has stopped and time has ceased to march forward. If we don't have patience, we simply won't make it. Jesus Christ needed patience when He walked on this earth, so once again we can turn to His example to help us. Just as Christ found special strength and endurance to deal with His trials, we can find the same if we will remember to turn to Him. We wait, but we never wait alone, and time passes just a bit quicker when we have someone to wait with.

April 1

But let patience have her perfect work, that ye may be perfect and entire, wanting nothing (James 1:4).

Wouldn't it be wonderful if there were a magic wand that we could wave, and suddenly the pounds would melt from our flesh and we would be the perfect weight? I know of no one who would choose the rigors and demands of a diet over a magic wand. Unfortunately, there are no magic wands, and the only way we can lose weight is to set ourselves to the task — body, mind, and spirit. We need to ask God's help, that we might remain committed to the task no matter how long it takes. When we call on the Lord, He will grant us the patience we so badly need.

Today's thought: The longer the wait, the less the weight!

April 2

For ye have need of patience, that, after ye have done the will of God, ye might receive the promise (Hebrews 10:36).

It seemed like forever before any weight came off. Gerri had cut way back on her food intake and exercised daily. It had been frustrating to step up on the scales day after day to find no real change. She stuck with the diet despite her despair, and now four weeks into the program it was paying off. People were beginning to notice the difference in her. What had seemed so painfully slow, one pound every few days, had finally added up, and she was thrilled. Waiting a little while had paid off, waiting a little more didn't seem nearly as hard.

Today's thought: I can take this diet one day at a time!

April 3

To every thing there is a season, and a time to every purpose under the heaven (Ecclesiastes 3:1).

There are times in our lives when a diet may be easier than at other times. In times of stress or tragedy, it may be impossible for us to lose weight. Diets take concentration and commitment. Things may come up to cause us to fall away from our diets, but we need to get started again as soon as possible. Just because we fail once doesn't mean we will fail every time. Pray for God's help and guidance. He will be faithful to help us through the tough times and the times we fail. God will make our way easier through His companionship and comfort.

Today's thought: There is no better time to diet than right now!

April 4

Rest in the Lord, and wait patiently for him: fret not thyself because of him who prospereth in his way, because of the man who bringeth wicked devices to pass (Psalms 37:7).

Is there anything worse than skinny people who act as if dieting were no big deal? It is so difficult to hear others criticize our efforts when they have absolutely no idea what we are going through. However, we need to understand that the comments of those who don't understand us really shouldn't affect us. The Lord loves us as we are, and He truly does understand the struggles we grapple with. He has compassion on His children, and He will deal with those who are cruel or unthinking in their dealings with us. Listen to the Lord, not to others who don't know us nearly as well.

Today's thought: Beware skinny people with fat mouths!

April 5
And the peace of God, which passeth all understanding, shall keep your hearts and minds through Christ Jesus (Philippians 4:7).

Leah was still terribly overweight. She had tried dozens of diets, none of which had made an impact. She attended church regularly, and she prayed continually for God to help her with her problem. She realized that she wasn't ready deep down inside, so she often ignored the voice of her conscience and the comfort of her prayers. Leah lived from day to day asking God's forgiveness and resolving to try harder in the future. She told her friends, "When I'm ready, I know God will be there, and I know He will help me lose all the weight I need to."

Today's thought: Lord, make me ready to lose weight!

April 6
I waited patiently for the Lord; and he inclined unto me, and heard my cry (Psalms 40:1).

Leah was not the kind of woman to just make excuses. When she said that God would help her when she was ready to let Him, she wasn't just copping out. A day came when Leah really needed and wanted to lose weight, and she did it. Though it was hard, Leah stuck to her diet, and she gave most of the credit to God. She had lived for years wishing that she could be thin. Only after trying and failing many times was she able to succeed. Waiting on the Lord can be tiring and defeating. However, no one knows us like God does, and if we can wait, He will always do what is best for us.

Today's thought: Our best effort will always include God.

April 7
I, therefore, the prisoner of the Lord, beseech you that ye walk worthy of the vocation wherewith ye are called, with all lowliness and meekness, with long-suffering, forbearing one another in love (Ephesians 4:1, 2).

Temper: It seems that the longer you diet, the shorter it gets. Keeping control of our temper is one of the harder parts of dieting. We feel everyone has some word of advice on what we ought to do differently, that no one really understands what we're going through, and no one appreciates all that we do without. It's no wonder we find ourselves a little short-tempered at times. That's when we need to turn to the source of all patience and peace. If Christ is allowed to rule in our hearts, we will find a new depth of tolerance and forbearance.

Today's thought: Losing weight is no excuse for losing patience!

April 8
For it is God which worketh in you both to will and to do of his good pleasure (Philippians 2:13).

Jeff made his living as a night watchman at a large company. He sat for hours at a console that housed a bank of television screens. For his efforts, he pulled a sizable paycheck. Many of Jeff's friends criticized him for getting so much for doing nothing. His reply, "Hey, if they're willing to pay it, why shouldn't I get it?"

Too often people look for ways of getting something for nothing. As God's children, we should always be looking for ways to be the best people we can be, not cutting corners, but committing ourselves to the pursuit of God's pleasure.

Today's thought: Today I will be the best dieter I can be!

April 9
For that which I do I allow not: for what I would, that do I not; but what I hate, that do I (Romans 7:15).

The lament of dieters everywhere: "But what I hate, that I do!" Then, after doing what we have vowed not to do, we turn the hate inward, and we are forced to deal with so much guilt. Why does dieting have to be so hard? Why can't we ever seem to have enough willpower to deal with all the temptations? The harder we try, the harder it gets. It's enough to drive a sane person crazy and a saint to sin. Praise God that He understands us so well and is ready to pick us up when we fall and set us back on the proper path. God is patient with us when we most need Him to be.

Today's thought: I will avoid the things I know I should not do!

April 10
Be still, and know that I am God: I will be exalted among the heathen, I will be exalted in the earth (Psalms 46:10).

Whenever food comes into my mind and I have the strongest urges to cheat on my diet, I just close my eyes, clear my head, and try to think of all the wonderful blessings God has given me. I ask God to help me, and then I wait very quietly for Him to answer my humble plea. God has never failed me. In some of the toughest situations, I feel His gentle presence, and my hunger and desire leave me. In the quiet times of our lives God comes the closest, because we do not shove Him aside with our other concerns. Call upon God, then wait. He will come.

Today's thought: If I keep my mouth shut, food can't get in!

April 11

And Jesus being full of the Holy Ghost returned from the Jordan, and was led by the Spirit into the wilderness, being forty days tempted of the devil. And in those days he did eat nothing: and when they were ended, he afterward hungered (Luke 4:1, 2).

Forty days without food. The thought boggles the mind. And yet, Jesus was able to do it. Though we are not Jesus, we do have the same source of comfort and strength as Jesus did: the Holy Spirit. If we will concern ourselves with filling up with the Holy Spirit, then we will not have so much time to fill up with other things. Just as Jesus was sustained through the forty days, we also will be sustained by the Spirit of the living, loving God.

Today's thought: Filling up with the Holy Spirit satisfies, and it isn't fattening!

April 12

Put on therefore, as the elect of God, holy and beloved, bowels of mercies, kindness, humbleness of mind, meekness, longsuffering (Colossians 3:12).

In centuries past, people went without food in order to break their willful spirits. Certain individuals knew they were too concerned with worldly things, and they wanted to humble themselves, so they went without food. A person who hungers loses conceit and cockiness very quickly. God wants us to have a spirit of lowliness and meekness. He wants us to shape our wills to His, and He wants us to be patient in all that we do. Dieting makes us very dependent. We are vulnerable, and we need someone to lean on. Thankfully, we have the Lord to lean on, who will bear our full weight, and never let us down.

Today's thought: I'd rather put on patience than put on weight!

April 13

And the word of the Lord came unto him, saying, Arise, get thee to Zarephath, which belongeth to Zidon, and dwell there: behold, I have commanded a widow woman there to sustain thee (1 Kings 17:8, 9).

Consider the prophet Elijah. The Lord told him to go to the town of Zarephath, where he was to wait for further guidance from God. Elijah waited there three years before the word came! How many of us would have such patience? Our dieting period often seems long, but in comparison with what so many others have had to go through, the time is really quite short. Committed people have always found a special source of patience and courage to get them through any situation. The source of their remarkable faith is the Lord, who makes all things possible.

Today's thought: I will make a little last a long, long time!

April 14

Let not your heart be troubled: ye believe in God, believe also in me (John 14:1).

The days will come when we question whether or not we will ever lose the weight we want to. Frustration can set in, and when it does, it makes us feel like such failures. Jesus' disciples found themselves feeling like failures at times in their lives. It was on those occasions that Jesus offered them the most comfort. Jesus understood human nature perfectly, and He came to let us know everything will work out fine. Turn to Christ when feelings of failure get strong. Our Lord of love and peace will not let us feel badly for long. His love truly conquers all.

Today's thought: True belief brings real relief!

April 15

. . . put off concerning the former conversation the old man, which is corrupt according to the deceitful lusts (Ephesians 4:22).

Fat people aren't bad people. Sometimes we feel inferior just because we happen to be overweight. It doesn't matter whether we're a few pounds over or a lot of pounds overweight, when we're too

46

heavy, it makes us feel bad. Obesity isn't a sin in itself, but often it is the result of sin. Gluttony, sloth, laziness; these things can lead to obesity, and they are sinful behaviors. When we decide to put off these wrong behaviors, we set ourselves on the path that pleases God. Change takes time, but the rewards are always worth the effort.

Today's thought: There's more to a new me than just losing weight.

April 16
Knowing this, that the trying of your faith worketh patience (James 1:3).

When you get really serious about losing weight, you have no alternative but to develop patience. There are no safe, quick ways to lose a lot of weight. It takes time. The body takes a long time to build up, and it takes a long time to wear down. However, the person who sticks with her diet will be amazed to find that the longer it's adhered to, the easier it gets. A time comes when the diet is no big deal. In many cases, people find they prefer their diet to their former way of eating. Patience is an elusive trait, but once it is attained, it is its own reward.

Today's thought: Patience would be a lot easier if it didn't take so long to get.

April 17
For our conversation is in heaven; from whence also we look for the Saviour, the Lord Jesus Christ (Philippians 3:20).

After Michelle promised Susan she would diet with her, she immediately began to regret it. All Susan did was talk about food. Susan had a one-track mind, and she made dieting so much harder for Michelle. Michelle constantly tried to change the direction of their conversations, but Susan always managed to bring the topic back to food. Finally, Michelle told Susan that if she didn't stop, she would no longer be able to be a diet partner with her. The two worked together and found that with some effort, they could steer clear of caloric conversation.

Today's thought: Lord, turn my mind away from the pleasures of my tummy!

April 18
Better is the end of a thing than the beginning thereof: and the patient in spirit is better than the proud in spirit (Ecclesiastes 7:8).

47

It doesn't take a genius to agree that the end of a diet is a lot better than the beginning. Oh, how wonderful it will be to finally reach the goal we set for ourselves, to finish this time of trial, temptation, and struggle! The Lord rejoices when we triumph in the pursuits of our everyday lives. He longs to see us happy and fulfilled. Pray to the Lord that He might bring you to the finish of your weight-loss program. He is faithful to stand beside us, granting the patience we need in all situations so we might finish victorious. Praise the Lord!

Today's thought: This day means I am one day closer to the end of my diet!

April 19

And it shall be said in that day, Lo, this is our God; we have waited for him and he will save us: this is the Lord; we have waited for him, we will be glad and rejoice in his salvation (Isaiah 25:9).

Barry was a clock-watcher. Instead of occupying himself in activities that would help the time pass more quickly, Barry chose to do nothing. He waited for things to happen, and as a result, he found himself continually nervous and anxious. Barry was never satisfied with the normal course of events. If we approach our diets with the same attitude as Barry, they will be torture for us. Ask God to help channel our attention to other things. Take control and find ways to get the mind on other things. When we wait patiently, engaged in things that are interesting and enjoyable, then we will find the wait is so much shorter.

Today's thought: There are a lot of things more interesting than food!

April 20

See then that ye walk circumspectly, not as fools, but as wise, redeeming the time, because the days are evil (Ephesians 5:15, 16).

A friend of mine always said, "If we would only spend time doing what we know we should, there wouldn't be any time left over to do the things we know we shouldn't." Simple truth, but hard truth to follow. When we diet, it is helpful to engage in activities that will prevent us from having the time to eat or even think about food. One person I knew joined a number of volunteer organizations, just so he would be too busy to eat all the time. We need to redeem the time that we spend in fattening endeavors, and turn instead to activities that are pleasing to God.

Today's thought: The busier I keep myself, the thinner I get!

April 21
Woe unto you that are full! for ye shall hunger. Woe unto you that laugh now! for ye shall mourn and weep (Luke 6:25).

As Christians, we need to keep in mind that we live in a world of terrible inequality. While we have the opportunities to overeat and overindulge, many people have no such chances. So many people starve. It is surely humbling to realize that much of our obesity comes from living in a culture where we can have pretty much all we want. The Lord Jesus Christ chastized the people of His day who were filled with the good things of life, because they ignored their brothers and sisters who had nothing. As we diet and feel the hunger in our stomachs, we are more aware of the feelings of our neighbors around the world who do not have enough to eat.

Today's thought: Make me less, Lord: less body, less selfishness, less ego!

April 22
Therefore I say unto you, Take no thought for your life, what ye shall eat, or what ye shall drink; nor yet for your body, what ye shall put on. Is not the life more than meat, and the body than raiment? (Matthew 6:25.)

When I began to diet, I realized how much of my time was spent with something to eat or drink in my hands. Before the diet, I had something in one hand or the other almost all the time. I used to spend a lot of time thinking about where I would eat, what I would eat, and how much I would eat. Food was an idol in my life. How foolish it is to live like that! There are so many things in life that are more important. Spend time in prayer and contemplation, asking the Lord to open the eyes of your heart to all the wonderful things you have missed for so long.

Today's thought: I want my life to be much more than food and drink!

April 23
Stand fast therefore in the liberty wherewith Christ hath made us free, and not be entangled again with the yoke of bondage (Galatians 5:1).

Patience gained during the diet is something well worth holding onto after the diet ends. How many people have lamented that they lost weight only to gain it back again. It is so silly to allow such a thing to happen. We struggle so hard to take weight off, why would we ever let it find a home on us again? Dieting frees us from the imprisonment of a fleshy jail. Once free from that, we should never return. Ask the Lord for strength and determination, so that once we liberate ourselves from fat, we may not be taken prisoner again!

Today's thought: I will not stand for slavery to flesh and fat!

April 24
Neither give place to the devil (Ephesians 4:27).

Satan would have us be much less than we have been created to be. He tempts us to gluttony and greed, then makes us feel weak and unworthy. He tries and tests us a thousand ways, and the harder we try to resist, the harder he works to thwart us. The only way to stand firm against the devil is to enlist the power of the Almighty God. Whereas Satan may have a field day with his human foes, he has no effects against God. When we give in to the temptation to indulge, we are really giving in to the plan of the devil to turn us from God. Follow the Lord at all times, and the devil will flee from you.

Today's thought: Chocolate cake is nothing but devil's food!

April 25
For I reckon that the sufferings of this present time are not worthy to be compared with the glory which shall be revealed in us (Romans 8:18).

Long-distance runners say they always keep the finish line in their mind's eye. The goal is the important thing. The runner who loses sight of the finish line is lost. In a like fashion, the dieter who loses sight of a newer, thinner self is lost. Diets are worth every effort we give them, though there are many times when that fact slips from our minds. The Apostle Paul found great strength in times of suffering by remembering that those who are faithful receive glory in the age to come. If we will keep our thoughts on the reward to come, our diets will be much easier.

Today's thought: I can suffer today for a new me tomorrow!

April 26
In every thing give thanks: for this is the will of God in Christ Jesus concerning you (1 Thessalonians 5:18).

It's easy to be thankful when we have everything we want or need. It's when we're forced to do without that thankfulness becomes difficult. Giving thanks for the opportunity to do without our daily bread is sometimes very, very hard. Yet, God is sure to help us when we need help the most. When we feel weak or hungry or unhappy, He will stand beside us and give us comfort. We're lucky to have God to rely on. Be thankful for the love and care of our Lord. In all things praise Him. When we learn to be thankful in our need, we are all the more thankful in our abundance.

Today's thought: If it is my heart's desire to be thin, God will help me!

April 27

Wait on the Lord: be of good courage, and he shall strengthen thine heart: wait, I say, on the Lord (Psalms 27:14).

There will be days when everything seems useless and impossible. The temptation to give up will be almost overwhelming. It is in those times of total desperation that we need to cry out to the Lord. The Lord truly will strengthen the hearts of those who call upon Him. The periods of despair will pass; the temptations will pass. What will never pass away is the loving support of God. He stands beside those who put their trust and faith in Him. Call out to God in the tough times. Rejoice with Him when the times are easy. Wait on the Lord, and He will bless your life!

Today's thought: As the wait goes on, the weight comes off!

April 28

If ye shall ask any thing in my name, I will do it (John 14:14).

A man asked help from his brothers, and they had no time. He turned to his children, and they had too many others things to do. He tried his friends, but they were all away. Feeling lonely and alone, he knelt down and prayed. Why is it that we turn to God only after all our other options are closed? God has promised to give us the desires of our hearts, and yet we seek them in a hundred other places. We need to make God our first choice, not our last. Keep the Lord first in your heart, first in your mind, and first in all you do and say. You'll be amazed what it can do for you!

Today's thought: A new me is mine for the asking!

April 29

And a woman having an issue of blood twelve years, which had spent all her living upon physicians, neither could be healed of any, came behind Him, and touched the border of his garment: and immediately her issue of blood stanched (Luke 8:43, 44).

How can we seriously feel sorry for ourselves when so many people have so little? Certainly, dieting produces discomfort, but it's very slight. We shouldn't let ourselves get carried away, making our diets a bigger deal than they need to be. However, the good news is, if God can take care of the really big things in life, He will have no trouble helping us through the trial of our diet. God gives good things to those who go out of their way to make Him part of their lives. Reach out to touch the hand of the Lord, and He will reach down to lift us above the struggles we face in life.

Today's thought: The touch of the Lord makes all things fine!

April 30

Behold, we count them happy which endure. Ye have heard of the patience of Job, and have seen the end of the Lord; that the Lord is very pitiful, and of tender mercy (James 5:11).

The end may not be in sight yet, but it's there somewhere. Ask the Lord for patience to make it work out. Job was beset by dozens of terrible afflictions, yet he kept his faith and his patience. He is a wonderful example for those of us who are dealing with the ordeal of a long diet. The Lord doesn't want us to suffer, even in small ways. When we diet, we open ourselves to a long, hard road of discomfort and struggle. Having the Lord on our side makes the struggle easier and the discomfort manageable. Job knew that as long as he had his faith, he had everything he needed to get by. The same is true for us today.

Today's thought: Patience makes the fast pass faster!

MAY
Faith

Faith is the foundation on which we build all our dreams, plans, and hopes. Nothing can be accomplished apart from faith. When we diet we need a deep and abiding faith in both ourselves and our Lord. If we fail to believe in ourselves, we might as well not even try to lose weight. Self-confidence and assurance is vital for success. When we find we have too much self-doubt, then we need to turn to the source of all faith: Jesus Christ, our Lord. Christ is the finest example of a faith-filled person we can find. Christ was able to face unbelievable trials because of the enormous faith He had in God. Through the gift of His Holy Spirit, we, too, can rely on this special faith. The faith of the Lord will never fail, nor will it decrease. Believe in the power of the Almighty God, and He will raise you up so you cannot be defeated.

May 1
Jesus said unto him, If thou canst believe, all things are possible to him that believeth (Mark 9:23).

All my friends said they didn't think I could do it. They watched me stuff myself so many times; they didn't think I had any self-control at all. I showed them. I knew in my heart I could make it. Sure, it was tough, but I'm no quitter. When the going got the toughest, it just made me more determined to lose the weight. The key is to believe in yourself. God believes in us, even though we don't always deserve His trust. If God can believe in us, then who are we to do otherwise? Pray for God's assurance, and you will find more than enough faith to make it through.

Today's thought: God believes in me!

May 2
And we know that all things work together for good to them that love God, to them who are the called according to his purpose (Romans 8:28).

Ed didn't really know what made him decide to try to take weight off, but now he was glad. His doctor had discovered an irregular heartbeat, and he told Ed to be thankful that he didn't have to carry around so much weight anymore, or his poor heart just wouldn't be able to bear the load. Ed secretly thanked the Lord for helping him out. No matter what had motivated Ed to lose, by doing so he had saved his own life. It was ironic, but Ed always knew that God makes all things work out for the best. After this, no one could ever convince him differently!

Today's thought: My diet may be the best idea God's had all day!

May 3

He that chastiseth the heathen, shall not he correct? he that teacheth man knowledge, shall not he know? (Psalms 94:10.)

Jill watched the television program to see the author of a diet plan she wanted to try. She settled in, hoping to be inspired by the man who had helped millions lose weight. When he came on, her heart sank. The man must have weighed three hundred pounds! How could you be inspired by someone who couldn't even practice what he preached? She had really hoped that at long last she had found a winner. Every time Jill put her faith in some new fad, it always seemed to fall apart. Jill guessed her mother was right: The only source worthy of her faith was Christ. Perhaps He really could help where everyone else had failed.

Today's thought: Following fads is frustrating and foolish!

May 4

He that handleth a matter wisely shall find good: and whoso trusteth in the Lord, happy is he (Proverbs 16:20).

Ben couldn't believe all the people he was talking with. They all wanted to lose weight overnight! None of them seemed to be looking at any practical programs. They had all latched on to crash diets with pills and books and foolish promises of miraculous results. Ben sat down and worked out a practical diet that he could live with, so that once he lost weight (and he realized it would take some time), he could stick with the diet and avoid putting the weight back on. When he said his prayers that night, he put in a special request for some common sense for his friends.

Today's thought: Trust is a must for weight to abate!

May 5

But without faith it is impossible to please him: for he that cometh to God must believe that he is, and that he is a rewarder of them that diligently seek him (Hebrews 11:6).

Denny looked at the enormous jigsaw puzzle with a gleam in his eye. "This is my puzzle, and I'm going to do it all by myself. Nobody else can touch it!" Denny worked at the puzzle long and hard, but grew frustrated as he couldn't get the pieces to work. Finally, in despair, Denny ran to his father and asked him to come make some of the pieces fit.

We cannot afford to enter into our diets with the attitude that we don't need help. Like Denny, we will find that we just can't do it by ourselves. Praise God that He is there for us when we come seeking His help!

Today's thought: I don't have to face my diet by myself.

May 6

That the trial of your faith, being much more precious than of gold that perisheth, though it be tried with fire, might be found unto praise and honour and glory at the appearing of Jesus Christ (1 Peter 1:7).

When the heavy-duty drearies set in, it is easy to question whether you believe in anything at all. Dieting is tedious, taxing, and trying. If there is a God, you may ask, why doesn't He just put us out of our misery? The Lord knows what we need, and He brings us through tough times so we might be made better for it. Just as gold is purified when subjected to intense heat, we are purified by our struggles. When we come through a situation, we are able to look back on it stronger than we were before. Trust the wisdom of the Lord, and He will reward you with faith and love.

Today's thought: I am made stronger every day that I diet!

May 7

For ye are all the children of God by faith in Christ Jesus (Galatians 3:26).

Sarah loved chocolate, but when her parents found out she was seriously allergic to it, they made sure she never got any. Sometimes when they were out, she would beg for some chocolate, but her parents never waivered. They allowed her other treats, but they were able to stand firm in their denial of chocolate out of the love they had for their daughter.

Our Lord watches all of us as beloved children. He wants us to have good things, but not things that are harmful to us. Overeating is indeed harmful, so we should not be surprised that God doesn't want us to do it.

Today's thought: Lord, help me avoid things that could harm me.

May 8
And they rose early in the morning, and went forth into the wilderness of Tekoa: and as they went forth, Jehoshaphat stood and said, Hear me, O Judah, and ye inhabitants of Jerusalem: Believe in the Lord your God, so shall ye be established; believe his prophets, so shall ye prosper (2 Chronicles 20:20).

Too many people fail in their endeavors because they have no backup system. When their own strength fails, they have nothing to fall back on. We Christians have a special advantage in the person of Jesus Christ. When we call out to Him, He is faithful to save us. When we believe in God, He establishes us and helps us attain the desire of our hearts. We need never doubt, as long as the power of the living Lord is on our side.

Today's thought: All my friends may rely on their own devices, but I will rely on the one who makes all things possible: Jesus Christ the Lord.

May 9
Jesus saith unto him, Thomas, because thou hast seen me, thou hast believed: blessed are they that have not seen, and yet have believed (John 20:29).

Too many of us suffer from Missouri disease. Missourians are noted for their skepticism, and that is why Missouri is known as the "show me" state. We look for some kind of impressive, spectacular sign. If we don't get it, then we disregard the source. God doesn't work through flashy signs and gimmicks. God works quietly and intimately, and He works His will in His own time. We may not always see the results when we want to, but relax; the Lord is at work, and we need have no fear that He will let us down.

Today's thought: The Lord is helping me, whether I can sense it or not.

May 10

And Jesus said unto them, Because of your unbelief: for verily I say unto you, If ye have faith as a grain of mustard seed, ye shall say unto this mountain, Remove hence to yonder place: and it shall remove; and nothing shall be impossible unto you (Matthew 17:20).

Too often we miss the point of the mustard seed. We think quantity of faith is the determining factor in getting our hearts' desires. Quantity has nothing to do with it. Jesus used the mustard seed to show that we all have at least that much faith, and if we will learn to employ it, we will see miraculous things happen in our lives. Because of our lives in Christ, nothing is impossible for us, including our diets.

Today's thought: If I can remove mountains, then I can remove pounds!

May 11

For whatsoever is born of God overcometh the world: and this is the victory that overcometh the world, even our faith (1 John 5:4).

When Jesus faced the devil in the wilderness, He was weak and hungry. He had fasted long and hard, and He would have given anything to be able to break that fast. Bread is a great temptation to a starving man. Yet, Jesus refused to give in to the temptations of the devil. No matter how enticing Satan was, Jesus was able to resist him. By resisting the devil, Jesus overcame him, and in so doing, He overcame the world and all it could offer Him. We, too, can overcome the world by having faith in the one who has already triumphed. No temptation on earth can bring us down, because we follow the one who overcame the whole world.

Today's thought: I will turn to Jesus whenever I need a faith lift!

May 12

For we are saved by hope: but hope that is seen is not hope: for what a man seeth, why doth he yet hope for? (Romans 8:24).

Gwen stopped by the dress shop every few days to look at the gown she had picked out. Though it was a couple of sizes smaller than she wore, she dreamed of the time she could fit into it. It was a perfect gown. She could visualize in her mind's eye how stunning she would look in it. For the next month, Gwen stuck to a strict diet and made her dream a reality. She lost the two sizes and bought the dress she wanted so badly.

We need our dreams, hopes, and plans to make it through our diets. Hope helps us bolster our faith and makes our dreams come true.

Today's thought: Hoping helps believing!

May 13

That ye be not slothful, but followers of them who through faith and patience inherit the promises (Hebrews 6:12).

Beverly held a support group at the church every Tuesday morning. Bev had been enormous before she began her diet, and to the amazement of the entire congregation, she had lost two hundred pounds. After losing her weight, Beverly had determined to help others in their fights to lose weight. Many people found help in turning to Beverly, because they knew she could sympathize with what they were experiencing. Other people had little use for Bev, because her way of losing weight was too demanding. Being Christian often means taking the hard way, but the hard way always offers us the greatest rewards.

Today's thought: Help me to benefit from the faith of others!

May 14

And he said unto her, Daughter, be of good comfort: thy faith hath made thee whole; go in peace (Luke 8:48).

When all is said and done, the determining factor in our diet is going to be our frame of mind. No one loses weight who doubts he can do it. The mind is a tricky thing, and it will tell us time and again that there is no way we can hope to succeed. It will create all kinds of monsters for us to overcome, and defeating them is not easy. Only the person who is mentally and spiritually prepared stands a chance of overcoming. When we truly believe in ourselves and our Lord, then we can go in peace, knowing that nothing on earth can get the better of us.

Today's thought: God is bigger than any craving my mind and stomach can come up with!

May 15

And immediately Jesus stretched forth his hand, and caught him, and said unto him, O thou of little faith, wherefore didst thou doubt? (Matthew 14:31.)

Peter asked the Lord to allow him to walk on the water. Seeing his Master walking on the waves caused Peter to wish to do likewise. However, once he began his walk, he found himself sinking and afraid. What did the Lord do at this sign of unbelief? Did He allow Peter to sink? Of course not! So long as Jesus is nearby, we need never fear for our lives. Jesus Christ reaches out His hand to us when we get in over our heads. Though He wants us to develop unshakable faith, He is forgiving and loving, and He lifts us up when we are too weak to stand up on our own.

Today's thought: Thank the Lord that Christ holds me up whem I'm most down!

May 16

Confess your faults one to another, and pray one for another, that ye may be healed. The effectual fervent prayer of a righteous man availeth much (James 5:16).

The group began every week by admitting all their transgressions. Having to admit all the wrongs that were done really helped act as a deterrent during the week. It was embarrassing to tell people about the things you shouldn't have eaten, even though they were all friends. What really made a difference was the period of prayer that ended each session. What a source of strength and courage! The group was the best thing Janet had ever gotten into. Dieting was almost a joy when it was done with such good friends. Sharing the experience helped Janet make her diet a success.

Today's thought: Confession is good for the soul and for the diet!

May 17

For by grace are ye saved through faith; and that not of yourselves: it is the gift of God (Ephesians 2:8).

Jerry was so confident. He knew he could lose weight if he would only knuckle down and try. But it seems that no matter how determined he got, something came up to thwart him. Whenever friends tried to help him, he told them to leave him alone; he was going to make it on his own.

How sad that some people try to do everything by themselves. It is good to believe in yourself, but not when that self-belief causes you to be less than you can be. Believe in God. Put your faith there. Whatever you find you cannot do, remember that God can do it.

Today's thought: Thank God for the gift of determination!

May 18

For therein is the righteousness of God revealed from faith to faith: as it is written, The just shall live by faith (Romans 1:17).

Jean had gone to church for years and had always known she was welcome there. Barbara attended a church across town from Jean's, and she was beginning to think it just wasn't right for her anymore. Both women saw each other at an exercise class that met on Monday mornings. One morning Barbara lamented about her disillusionment with her church, and Jean invited her to come to church with her on Sunday morning. Barbara immediately felt at home in Jean's church, and the two women developed a strong relationship. Faith met faith at an exercise/weight-loss class, and a beautiful friendship was born.

Today's thought: I will use my diet for the glory of God.

May 19

He that believeth and is baptized shall be saved; but he that believeth not shall be damned (Mark 16:16).

It is so easy to be tossed back and forth in our commitment to our diets. One day they seem worth the effort, and the next they seem like such a drag. It feels like they will never end, and nothing we do makes the time pass any further. The sad fact is, it is up to us. If we stick to our diets, we'll lose weight. If we cheat, then we can't expect to lose. Just as the Christian who believes receives the eternal reward and those who don't believe will have no part in it, dieters who remain faithful reap the reward, while those who lose heart receive nothing.

Today's thought: In dieting, the biggest winner is the biggest loser!

May 20

If ye abide in me, and my words abide in you, ye shall ask what ye will, and it shall be done unto you (John 15:7).

"I don't really believe in God. I keep asking Him for things, and I never get them. I want new clothes, a decent car, and I'm tired of working. I go to church regularly, and I pray all the time. The Bible says that if I ask for anything in God's name I'll get it. I think it's a bunch of hogwash."

Too many people think all they have to do is ask, and God will shower them with wealth and luxuries of life. God does indeed want us to have good things, but He tells us that we must ask for things with a Christlike mind. We need to ask ourselves, "Would Christ ask for this!" Ask in the Spirit of Jesus the Christ, and God will bless you richly.

Today's thought: I need God's help to ask for the right things.

May 21
Now faith is the substance of things hoped for, the evidence of things not seen (Hebrews 11:1).

Jimmy wanted the bicycle so badly he could taste it. His mother and father had told him to save for it, and they would help him buy it. He remembered his father saying, "If it's important enough to you, you'll be surprised how easy it is to save your money." He hoped this was true, because he sure wanted the bike.

If we want to lose weight badly enough, we'll be surprised how easily we can stick to our diets. When the goal is great enough, we find sufficient supplies of faith and determination to overcome any temptation.

Today's thought: I want to be a substantial person without having a substantial body!

May 22
Hast thou faith? have it to thyself before God. Happy is he that condemneth not himself in that thing which he alloweth (Romans 14:22).

Face it: You're going to give in a few times along the way. You know it, I know it, and most importantly, God knows it. As human beings, we have to face the fact that there are times we are very weak. Too many people condemn themselves and find it hard to go on. That's nonsense. When we fall down and indulge in a special treat we should not have, we should repent of the transgression but not of the happiness the treat gave us. Those things that fatten us are good, and we like them a lot. There is nothing wrong with liking them, and there is nothing to be ashamed of in falling back now and again.

Today's thought: If God thinks I'm forgivable, who am I to argue?

May 23

But we had the sentence of death in ourselves, that we should not trust in ourselves, but in God which raiseth the dead (2 Corinthians 1:9).

Alice walked ahead of me in the lunch line. As we moved along, Alice would hesitate, reach out her hand, then pull it back. After she had done this a couple of times, I noticed that she had three letters written on the back of her hand: GIW. I asked her what they meant. She looked at me and said, "God Is Watching. I figure if I keep reminding myself of that, it will keep me out of trouble."

When we cannot trust ourselves, it is good to know there is someone to trust who will not let us down: Jesus Christ.

Today's thought: Watch me closely Lord. I'm hungry, and I'm weak.

May 24

Now the just shall live by faith: but if any man draw back, my soul shall have no pleasure in him (Hebrews 10:38).

Helen lamented that she couldn't lose weight, but she hardly ever tried. Oh, she would spend time with her friends talking about diets, and she would go to exercise class and sit on the side of the gym while her friends exercised, and she would buy diet sodas and TV dinners, but she would also buy coffee cakes and ice cream. The saddest thing about Helen was that she couldn't understand why her friends weren't sympathetic to her. Everyone, including God, will sympathize with us when we are giving it our best efforts. However, if we deal with losing weight like Helen, even God will have little patience with us.

Today's thought: Only fools think they fool God!

May 25

Therefore, my beloved brethren, be ye stedfast, unmovable, always abounding in the work of the Lord, forasmuch as ye know that your labour is not in vain in the Lord (1 Corinthians 15:58).

The Lord wants us to develop strong convictions. The best Christians are the ones who are unwavering in their faith. God will help us develop a lot of iron so we might become totally committed to whatever we set our minds to. As dieters, we need that kind of conviction. If we can stand firm in our resolve to lose weight, we can become examples of the power of God to change lives, physically as well as spiritually. When we commit our endeavors to the Lord, we raise them above personal goals and make them a part of our faith walk; a walk we never make alone.

Today's thought: Let my spirit be immovable, not my body!

May 26
Be ye therefore followers of God, as dear children (Ephesians 5:1).

As children of loving parents, we always knew they would do what was best for us: loving us, protecting us, providing for us, and teaching us. Our parents wanted us to be happy and fulfilled, and they sacrificed much so we could enjoy life. The Bible reminds us that our heavenly Father loves us even more than any earthly parent ever could. We should follow the wisdom of the Lord as children follow the loving guidance of their parents. God will keep us from those things we should not have, if we will only ask Him to. Include God in every aspect of your life, including your diet.

Today's thought: Let me be a *little* child of God!

May 27
So then faith cometh by hearing, and hearing by the word of God (Romans 10:17).

"How do I know that God will help me lose weight?"
The question comes up often, and there is only one response to give:
God will help us in every time of need, and He will never turn us away. That is something we just have to know by faith, and we bolster that faith by listening to the word of God: the Holy scriptures. God makes wonderful promises to His people, and He is faithful to keep each and every one. He will help us understand His will, if we will only allow Him to do it in His own time and His own way. Listen to the promises of God and receive faith.

Today's thought: I can't hear God if there's fat between my ears!

May 28
For which cause we faint not; but though our outward man perish, yet the inward man is renewed day by day (2 Corinthians 4:16).

63

It is interesting how we feel so much better about ourselves when we lose weight. As the fleshy part of our being diminishes, the spiritual part of us blossoms. As we decrease our body mass, we find that we unburden hidden parts of our being. We are renewed inside as we take care of the bodies we have been given by God. It is not a matter of being perfect, but of being the best we can possibly be. If we will only keep in mind that we are temples of the most high God, then we will be encouraged to do everything in our power to look and be the best that we are able.

Today's thought: As there is less of me, there is more of God!

May 29

Jesus answered and said unto them, Verily I say unto you, If ye have faith, and doubt not, ye shall not only do this which is done to the fig tree, but also if ye shall say unto this mountain, Be thou removed, and be thou cast into the sea; it shall be done (Matthew 21:21).

Most people like to feel they are in control of their lives. When they are manipulated or made to feel helpless, they rebel and fight with everything they can. Funny how many of the same people allow food to control them and never give it a thought. Christian people are people who refuse to be ruled by their passions. They ask themselves, "What would Jesus have me do and be?" rather than leaping into situations without any forethought. Christ should be the only ruler of our lives, and when we turn all power over to Him, miraculous things begin to happen.

Today's thought: The same power that withers figs can wither fat!

May 30

Above all, taking the shield of faith, wherewith ye shall be able to quench all the fiery darts of the wicked (Ephesians 6:16).

When we diet, we need protection. We really do. Dieting puts us in a very vulnerable position. We are weakened, frustrated, irritable, guilty, and a hundred other things that stir us up constantly. We need a shield to guard us from the onslaught of so many difficult emotions and feelings. The Lord provides us with the shield we need through faith. Believing in a God who cares for us and stands beside us is a great comfort and a very real help in our times of need. God will not let us struggle alone. He is our refuge, our shield against the worst our diets can do to us.

Today's thought: Oh, Lord, please protect me from me!

May 31

For I say, through the grace given unto me, to every man that is among you, not to think of himself more highly than he ought to think; but to think soberly, according as God hath dealt to every man the measure of faith (Romans 12:3).

There are three young men who found they were in need of help from their fathers. The first young man went to his father, but his father told him he didn't deserve any help. The second young man went to his father, but he was told he could have only so much help, then no more. The last young man went to his father, and he was given all the help he needed, and then some. The father let his son know that no matter how much he needed, he could always come to him. Our Father in heaven is like the third father. We need much help in getting through our diets, and we can know through faith that God will always be there to provide us with what we need.

Today's thought: The more I give up, the more God gives!

JUNE
Hope

In this day and age, we need to believe tomorrow will be better than today. It is imperative that we set goals, follow dreams, and strive to be more than we have in the past. When people live without hope, they cease to really live at all. Hope is the key to a full and happy life. Hope gives us something to look forward to. Hope puts meaning into our lives. Hope keeps us going when everything else is gone. Hope is one of the greatest powers we can tap into. As we fight to lose weight, hope needs to be one of our closest companions. Dieters must be hopeful people if they want to succeed, and Jesus Christ is the focus of our deepest hope. He alone can supply us with all the power we need to remain hopeful in tough situations. Call upon the Lord, and He will give you hope beyond reason. As long as we live in hope, we can count on being made conquerors alongside the one who conquers all so we might live: Jesus the Christ.

June 1
For now we see through a glass, darkly; but then face to face: now I know in part; but then shall I know even as also I am known (1 Corinthians 13:12).

One thing would really make dieting easier: Knowing what the results are actually going to look like. When we diet, we have to hold onto some image we have created in our own minds. Perhaps it is an image crafted from an old picture, or a memory of what we looked like so many years ago. Still, there is no tangible goal we can point to and say, "That is what I will look like when I lose weight." We have to live in hope of something we want, and hope can be scary. Ask God to help you. He will enable us to believe in what we imagine, even when we can't always see it in reality.

Today's thought: I'll know better why I'm dieting after I'm done!

June 2

Beloved, now are we the sons of God, and it doth not yet appear what we shall be: but we know that, when he shall appear, we shall be like him; for we shall see him as he is. And every man that hath this hope in him purifieth himself, even as he is pure (1 John 3:2, 3).

Sometimes we fool ourselves into believing that to be like Jesus means to act like Him or think like Him or pray like Him, and we ignore that we should try to look like Him, too. We don't know that Jesus was thin, but we can be confident that He was not overweight, because He preached moderation and denounced gluttony. He cared for Himself, and He called others to care for themselves, also. How wonderful it would be to be able to stand face-to-face with our Lord and to mirror Him in both His spiritual and physical perfection!

Today's thought: When people look at me, I want them to see Jesus!

June 3

For thou art my hope, O Lord God: thou art my trust from my youth (Psalms 71:5).

A friend of mine slipped into a well when he was a child, and all he remembers of the experience was praying to God and awaiting rescue. He recounts how he felt no fear because he knew God would get him out of his trouble. He placed his hope in the Lord, and he was not disappointed.

Being overweight can sometimes feel like being in the bottom of a deep, dark well, with no way out. But we do have a way out. The Lord is a lifeline and a Savior indeed. If we will place our trust in Him, He will be faithful to lift us out of the dark places and set us fully in the light.

Today's thought: Lift me from my well of obesity!

June 4

And hope maketh not ashamed; because the love of God is shed abroad in our hearts by the Holy Ghost which is given unto us (Romans 5:5).

There will be those days when we feel we're never going to lose any weight. No matter what we do, the pounds stick with us, and we begin to feel foolish for ever supposing we could lose weight.

We find ourselves ashamed for believing that we can lose weight and ashamed at having such defeatist thoughts. It's a very hard position to be in. Luckily, we never really have to feel ashamed of the things we try to do that are good and right. Even though we sometimes lose heart, we still have the love and support of the Lord, who will strengthen us and guide us through His Spirit.

Today's thought: I'm proud of what I'm trying to do!

June 5

Wherefore gird up the loins of your mind, be sober, and hope to the end for the grace that is to be brought unto you at the revelation of Jesus Christ (1 Peter 1:13).

Fighters have to prepare for their bouts in every way possible. They train for a long time, working toward physical perfection. They eat properly, they rest regularly, they follow the instructions of their trainers closely, and they psych themselves up. Psyching entails a preparation of the mind that equals the preparation of the body. Dieters need that kind of mental preparation. As the scripture says, we must "gird up the loins" of our minds. We are fighters against fatness, and the only way we can hope to be victorious is to prepare ourselves completely, day by day, in body, spirit, and mind.

Today's thought: I'm ready for a good fight against fat!

June 6

And it came to pass, when he was in a certain city, behold a man full of leprosy: who seeing Jesus fell on his face, and besought him, saying, Lord, if thou wilt, thou canst make me clean (Luke 5:12).

Being overweight can sometimes feel like having leprosy. Fatness sets us apart from others and makes us feel different. We feel like outcasts, rejected by our "thin is in" society. Our greatest hope comes to us through the power of the Lord, who is willing to help us in every way possible in our attempts to lose weight. Like the man full of leprosy, all we need do is stretch out our hands to Jesus, and He will make us clean. We do not have to live as outcasts, but are full members of the glorious family of our Lord, and He is waiting to welcome us.

Today's thought: Fitness, as well as cleanliness, is next to godliness.

June 7

And every man that hath this hope in him purifieth himself, even as he is pure (1 John 3:3).

One of the best side effects of dieting is the purging our bodies receive. Interestingly, our bodies function best when we eat less. We don't overload our systems, and therefore they work better. Our bodies get cleaned out, and we feel better. It is easy to forget that we are helping our bodies operate at peak efficiency, and that our dieting cleans our entire system. Few people would mind feeling great, and God wishes for all of us a healthy, happy life. He created our systems to maintain themselves, but they can only do so if we will respect them and care for them properly.

Today's thought: My body's in need of a good spring cleaning!

June 8

And when he was come into the house, the blind men came to him: and Jesus saith unto them, Believe ye that I am able to do this? They said unto him, Yea, Lord (Matthew 9:28).

Doubt is a killer. It kills our enthusiasm, our faith, our hope, our initiative, and our dedication. When we begin to doubt that we can succeed in our diet attempts, we lose the most vital ingredient for success. You have to believe. In scripture, Jesus often asked people if they believed He could do miracles. When they said yes, fantastic things happened, but when they said no, nothing much happened. We need to say yes to God and believe He will bless all of our attempts to lose weight. With God on our side, there is absolutely no reason for doubt to affect us at all.

Today's thought: I'll try to believe, so more pounds will leave.

June 9

And we desire that every one of you do shew the same diligence to the full assurance of hope unto the end: That ye be not slothful, but followers of them who through faith and patience inherit the promises (Hebrews 6:11, 12).

Dr. Davidson always had a policy with his patients who tried to lose weight. If he wanted them to lose twenty pounds, he told them they were to lose thirty. If they were to lose fifty pounds, he told them seventy-five. He knew that people would set their minds toward their goal, but that most of them would tire along the way.

To counteract that, he always set a goal that was beyond what was actually necessary. Though people did indeed tire before they reached the goal Dr. Davidson set, they did not give up before they reached the point they really needed to attain. Sustaining our energy for a diet is hard, but with the hand of God guiding us, we can make it.

Today's thought: The only thing I will give up is weight!

June 10

Whom having not seen, ye love; in whom, though now ye see him not, yet believing, ye rejoice with joy unspeakable and full of glory (1 Peter 1:8).

When it's all over, we can hardly believe we struggled so much. The reward of losing weight is so great that it wipes out all the bad memories along the way. We experience such a sense of triumph and joy, accomplishment and goodwill. We feel a power from within that helps us believe that anything is possible to us, if we will only have patience, courage, and commitment. God has made us conquerors, and He empowers us to do those things which we set our minds and hearts to. When we live life in hope of glories to come and pursue those glories with everything we have, the Lord will reward us and bless us richly.

Today's thought: I may not see it yet, but a new me is right around the corner!

June 11

Behold, the eye of the Lord is upon them that fear him, upon them that hope in his mercy; to deliver their soul from death, and to keep them alive in famine (Psalms 33:18, 19).

Hunger can be a terrible, terrible feeling. It is unbelievable that just being hungry can make us feel so sick and weak, but it does. We need to find ways to train our minds to ignore the pleasings of the stomach. We need to engage in activities that will occupy our minds and absorb us, so we won't think of the food we should not have. In days gone by, people used to carry a copy of the gospels with them, and whenever they felt tempted to do what they knew they should not do, they pulled out the Bible and read scriptures until the desire passed. God is a wonderful diversion to occupy ourselves with when temptations arise.

Today's thought: I'm not dying of hunger; it just feels that way!

June 12
But he answered and said unto them, An evil and adulterous generation seeketh after a sign; and there shall no sign be given to it, but the sign of the prophet Jonas (Matthew 12:39).

Everybody wants guarantees. Everyone wants an escape clause: Money back if not completely satisfied. Unfortunately, the world doesn't work that way all the time. Often, there are no guarantees. Sadly, many people approach their faith in Christ in a similar fashion. They don't want to believe unless there are guarantees. They want to have some sign that will remove all doubts. There are signs of God's goodness and glory all around us, but we ignore them all too often. God does not promise us that He will take all obstacles from our lives. Instead, He promises to stay with us and help us learn to conquer them. We need no sign: God is with us, and His love is forever.

Today's thought: Christ is all the guarantee of success I need!

June 13
And I heard a great voice out of heaven saying, Behold, the tabernacle of God is with men, and he will dwell with them, and they shall be his people, and God himself shall be with them, and be their God (Revelation 21:3).

Indeed, there is strength in numbers. When we stand alone, we are very vulnerable, and it is easy to give in to trial and temptation. When we stand with others who can relate to our situation, we find a special strength that allows us to cope. Our Lord put us on earth to live together; to draw upon the strength that comes through fellowship. We have fellowship with one another and with God. He is with us wherever we may be. By His presence, He turns our weakness into strength and helps us hang on through the tough times.

Today's thought: God makes my hopes reality!

June 14
But let us, who are of the day, be sober, putting on the breastplate of faith and love; and for an helmet, the hope of salvation (1 Thessalonians 5:8).

In battle, the helmet is one of the most important protections. Head wounds can be fatal, and so the helmet must be strong. No soldier would think of entering the fray without proper head protection. Thessalonians says that our Christian helmet is the hope of salvation. Christ gives us that helmet. Through the hope we have in Christ, we are protected and prepared to meet the challenges of our lives. Dieting is just one of those challenges, and without hope of success and completion, we are ill-equipped to meet that challenge. The greater our hope, the better our chance to lose weight.

Today's thought: Lord, give me a helmet which covers my mouth, too!

June 15
. . . Jesus Christ, by whom also we have access by faith into this grace wherein we stand, and rejoice in hope of the glory of God (Romans 5:1, 2).

Some days we just need to stop and congratulate ourselves on how far we've come. Perhaps there aren't a lot of outward signs of our diet yet. Perhaps we aren't even close to where we hope to be. Perhaps we still have a long way to go. That's okay. Sometimes we need to rejoice in the progress we've made in order to have the energy to keep on going. The Lord created in six days, and on the seventh He rested. In every endeavor, especially the difficult ones, we need a break to sit back and enjoy what we've done so far. Even if the beginnings are humble, we can feel good that we are devoted to doing something good for ourselves.

Today's thought: I'm better than I was yesterday, and I can't wait until tomorrow!

June 16
That by two immutable things, in which it was impossible for God to lie, we might have a strong consolation, who have fled for refuge to lay hold upon the hope set before us: which hope we have as an anchor of the soul, both sure and stedfast, and which entereth into that within the veil (Hebrews 6:18, 19).

When waters get choppy and the foul weather blows in, those who sail know enough to drop anchor so they won't be capsized or dashed onto the rocks. We can learn a lesson from that. As we fight to lose weight, we may find the weather a little foul and the waters a little choppy. Thank God that He is our anchor in all situations of stress and turmoil. If we remember to place our hopes in Him, He will protect us from the temptations and desires that threaten to sink our diets. Call upon the Lord, and He will answer you, and you will be saved.

Today's thought: God makes me immovable in my determination to lose weight!

June 17

Why art thou cast down, O my soul? and why art thou disquieted within me? hope thou in God: for I shall yet praise him, who is the health of my countenance, and my God (Psalms 42:11).

Our society would have us believe that the person who tries to do something is a failure unless he or she succeeds. Very little honor is awarded the person who gives it her best shot but falls short of the goal. How sad, for it is the person who does her very best who pleases God the most. When we decide to diet and we try to be as faithful to it as we can be, then we are victors in the eyes of the Lord. We need never grow discouraged when we don't lose weight, as long as we are doing the best job we can.

Today's thought: I judge myself harder than God does!

June 18

Watch ye therefore: for ye know not when the master of the house cometh, at even, or at midnight, or at the cockcrowing, or in the morning (Mark 13:35).

Diets need to be taken one day at a time. Each new day means a new diet. If yesterday's diet didn't work, it doesn't really matter. Whether we diet tomorrow or not doesn't matter, either. What does matter is today. Too often we get caught up thinking about all the things we haven't done or dreaming of all the things we ought to do, and we have no time to actually do the things we have set before us right now. God's people live in the present. They learn from the past and hope for the future, but they make the most of every single moment of every day. Live for today and see the miracles begin.

Today's thought: Today's diet will be a success!

June 19

When thou passest through the waters, I will be with thee; and through the rivers, they shall not overflow thee: when thou walkest through the fire, thou shalt not be burned; neither shall the flame kindle upon thee (Isaiah 43:2).

Diets are endurance tests. How long can we hope when we feel as if the end of our trial is nowhere in sight? There will be an end to our diets, even though we often can't see it. It is good to know that God is with us and He is there to listen to us and share with us throughout our diet. God will be faithful to turn every kind of bad situation to good use. God is the source of our hope. Even when we can't see an end, God will give us the strength and determination we need to succeed. We cannot be beaten in our diets as long as we place our hope in God.

Today's thought: I can always make it through just one more day!

June 20

Thus saith the Lord; Refrain thy voice from weeping, and thine eyes from tears: for thy work shall be rewarded, saith the Lord; and they shall come again from the land of the enemy. And there is hope in thine end, saith the Lord, that thy children shall come again to their own border (Jeremiah 31:16, 17).

Stephanie looked at the pictures from her wedding day. Had she really ever been that thin? How had the pounds found their way onto her body in such a few short years? She determined that she was going to return to her former figure by the end of the year. As a Christmas present to herself and her family, she was going to be able to wear her wedding dress once again. With a great sense of hope, Stephanie worked to her goal, and as subtly as the pounds had accumulated, they began to melt away. With the help of the Lord, we can always escape the enemy of fat and return to the land of fitness.

Today's thought: God helps me beat the fat foe!

June 21

Having therefore these promises, dearly beloved, let us cleanse ourselves from all filthiness of the flesh and spirit, perfecting holiness in the fear of God (2 Corinthians 7:1).

Barrie never felt good after stuffing himself. He felt weighted down and slow. He was grumpy and irritable. He usually felt sick. Still, when food was around, he couldn't help himself. Other people would watch him eat, and he could tell they thought it was a disgrace. What could he do? Nobody understood how hard it was for him. He wanted to lose weight and pass by second and third helpings, but he just didn't have the willpower. Too bad Barrie didn't have the support of good Christian friends and a commitment to sacrificing for God. With that kind of support, anyone can hope to lose weight.

Today's thought: There's no reason for me to face my diet alone!

June 22

And the Lord shall help them, and deliver them: he shall deliver them from the wicked, and save them, because they trust in him (Psalms 37:40).

Beth thought the program would never end. It had taken her years to control her weight, and it was still hard to be around scrumptious food for very long without overindulging. All through the evening, heavenly plates of food moved around the room. It was all Beth could do to resist. Whenever the temptation arose, she closed her eyes and quietly prayed to God for strength. It seemed like an eternity, but the evening finally ended, and she had somehow made it through. With a sigh of relief, she said a quick prayer of thanks as she walked to her car.

Today's thought: When I can't make it, God can!

June 23

Wherefore thou art no more a servant, but a son; and if a son, then an heir of God through Christ (Galatians 4:7).

Kerry knew God loved her when she was fat, but she felt His love so much more now that she was thin. She knew it had nothing to do with how much God really loved her, but with how much she loved herself. Now, she could look in the mirror without shame blushing her cheeks. Now, she could hold her head up and not worry about what other people thought of her. Once she had been a slave to her body. Now, she was free to be everything she wanted to be. She had once believed she would never be free of the weight that burdened her not only physically, but emotionally, too. God indeed worked wonders!

Today's thought: With God's help, I will be free from fat.

June 24

And the peace of God, which passeth all understanding, shall keep your hearts and minds through Christ Jesus (Philippians 4:7).

Promises. Every diet made promises, and they very rarely came through. Jenny had tried a dozen diets, each time putting her faith in their promises. Quietly, with tears in her eyes, she prayed for God's help. She wanted to lose weight so badly. As she prayed, she felt calm and hopeful. If only she could feel so peaceful when temptation raised its ugly head. Jenny vowed to try turning to God for help in the future instead of turning to more fad diets. Maybe God could do things for her that diet plans couldn't. She didn't really understand it. but she believed it was true.

Today's thought: If I turn to God, there's always hope!

June 25

Then shall we know, if we follow on to know the Lord: his going forth is prepared as the morning; and he shall come unto us as the rain, as the latter and former rain unto the earth (Hosea 6:3).

Carol went to a Christian prayer group with some skepticism. Gladys and Ann had started going, and they had immediately made great strides in their diets. Both women gave all the credit to God, but Carol wasn't convinced. She thought it sounded way too easy. Why would God do something for her that she ought to be able to do for herself? Carol wanted to believe, but she just couldn't quite believe that God would be interested enough in her weight problem to help her out. Too bad for Carol that she never realized how trustworthy the Lord is. If we put our faith in Him, He will be sure to help us.

Today's thought: No matter is too insignificant to bring to God!

June 26

For every creature of God is good, and nothing to be refused, if it be received with thanksgiving (1 Timothy 4:4).

Greg tried not to get discouraged, even though he gained back most of the weight he'd lost. This time it would be easier. He'd done it once; he could do it again. The first time had been so hard because he had such a low opinion of himself. His self-image had improved immensely, and he had the confidence he needed to know he could lose weight. Greg knew he was made in God's image, even if that image got hidden a little now and then. Knowing that he was loved made losing weight much easier. Greg was thankful that God loved him so. He could conquer anything, with God's help.

Today's thought: Good things come to those who believe they will!

June 27
Be of good courage, and he shall strengthen your heart, all ye that hope in the Lord (Psalms 31:24).

Gail's wedding day was getting close. She had vowed to lose fifty pounds by the time she got married. She was within ten pounds of her goal, but the last ten pounds were the hardest. She was so worried that she might not make it. She sat alone, looking at the dress, and then she bowed her head to pray. As she asked the Lord for help, she renewed her promise to do everything she could to lose the weight. Suddenly, deep inside, she knew she was going to make it. Everything she hoped for would work out, because the Lord was giving her the strength and courage she needed to succeed.

Today's thought: When God says it will work out, it works out!

June 28
Let us therefore come boldly unto the throne of grace, that we may obtain mercy, and find grace to help in time of need (Hebrews 4:16).

Jeffrey never wanted to put anybody out. Instead of asking for help, he would struggle along on his own. Often, Jeffrey didn't get anything accomplished because he refused to impose on anyone else.

Sometimes, we act that way with God. We ask ourselves why God would be interested in helping us solve our problems. The thing is, God wants us to come to Him with our heartfelt needs. We have been invited to come before the throne of grace, and that includes with our diets. When we're honest, we'll admit that we need help, and there is no greater source of help than God.

Today's thought: Our hope to lose weight becomes reality when we put our trust in God.

June 29

. . . I count all things but loss for the excellency of the knowledge of Christ Jesus my Lord: for whom I have suffered the loss of all things, and do count them but dung, that I may win Christ (Philippians 3:8).

A young man dreamed that he was standing before a table spread with a wide array of tantalizing foods. Beyond the table stood Jesus. The young man began eating the food, and he became completely engrossed in his consumption. When he finished, Jesus was gone, and he didn't know where to look to find Him.

Whenever we engage in gluttony of any kind, our attention is turned from Christ to our own selfish wants. There should be nothing more important in our lives than doing what is pleasing to God. He wants us to be the best we can possibly be. Food, and our love of food, should always take a second place to our love of the Lord.

Today's thought: Eating pleases me; dieting pleases God!

June 30

And let us not be weary in well doing: for in due season we shall reap, if we faint not (Galatians 6:9).

Gwen hadn't seen Ed in almost five years. When they had last been together, she had been very overweight. She had struggled and fought to lose over the years, and she was quite proud of what she had accomplished. She could hardly wait to see his reaction. That was one of the best things about losing weight: seeing the faces of old friends who could hardly recognize you. The looks she got made the fight worthwhile. Their disbelief made Gwen feel she'd performed a miracle. Good things truly did come to those who waited and stuck to their hope. God had blessed her a hundredfold.

Today's thought: What I lose today in weight will be gain in other ways tomorrow!

JULY
Perseverance

It is so difficult to be tested. We desire to please God and to succeed in our endeavors, but sometimes our quests seem too hard. It is easy to lose courage and enthusiasm. God understands how hard it is for us to do the things we know we ought to. He also understands that tough experiences are necessary in order for us to mature and develop in our faith. With God's help we can make it through anything. He gives us the strength to persevere. He encourages us when everything seems dark and hopeless. He promises that we will find great reward when we fight to hang on and not give up. Perseverance is truly a gift from God. It is given to us in order that we might exist in this world and one day overcome it. We please the Lord when we fight the good fight and strive to be the best people we can be. That includes taking care of the body we have been given, and nothing requires perseverance like dieting does.

July 1

When wisdom entereth into thine heart, and knowledge is pleasant unto thy soul; discretion shall preserve thee, understanding shall keep thee: That thou mayest walk in the way of good men, and keep the paths of the righteous (Proverbs 2:10, 11, 20).

Knowing what was right and doing what was right are completely different matters. Jessica knew she should lose weight, and she knew the way to do that was to cut back on what she was eating. The problem was that she didn't want to give up any of the foods she loved. She just wasn't committed enough. A friend of hers told her that she had all the knowledge she needed in her head, but none of it was in her heart. The reason she couldn't stick to her diet was that she didn't want to lose weight badly enough. When we find ourselves lacking the proper desire, we need to turn to the Lord, to ask His strength for doing what we know to be right.

Today's thought: Dieting is more than a matter of the mind. It's a matter of the heart!

July 2

In your patience possess ye your souls (Luke 21:19).

Arlene asked the Lord for just a little more patience. She looked at the clock. She had eaten lunch just three hours before, and now her stomach was telling her to eat again. She knew she really couldn't need food again so soon. She concentrated all her attention on the project she was working on and repeated again and again that she wasn't hungry. Before she knew it, she was finishing the project, her hunger had died down, and it was almost five o'clock. Quickly, Arlene thanked God for helping her hang on awhile. It wasn't nearly as hard to get by with God giving her strength and support.

Today's thought: Decide to control your stomach instead of letting it control you!

July 3

And ye shall be hated of all men for my name's sake: but he that endureth to the end shall be saved (Matthew 10:22).

Christ has a powerful lesson for those who choose to diet. Dieting makes us different, and it is never easy to be different. Being Christian made the disciples different, and they had to suffer many things for their difference. People who are different are often excluded by others. Sometimes they are even abused and persecuted for their differences. There was only one reason the disciples were able to persevere in their faith, and that was the presence of the Holy Spirit in their lives. That same Spirit can give us the power to be different and the strength to persevere, even through a tough diet.

Today's thought: Christ helps those who choose to be different!

July 4

Blessed is the man that endureth temptation: for when he is tried, he shall receive the crown of life, which the Lord hath promised to them that love him (James 1:12).

Christ allows us to declare a special kind of independence from the prison of obesity. Prisoners endure their captivity because they believe that they will one day find release. Through perseverance we earn the right to declare our independence from fat. God will stand with us as we fight for a healthier, more slender body.

His Holy Spirit will help us withstand the temptations of rich, fattening foods, and He promises to bless our efforts to do what is right and good. Let us celebrate the freedom from flesh that God will help us achieve.

Today's thought: Faith in Christ can lead to freedom from fat!

July 5

. . . We glory in tribulations also: knowing that tribulation worketh patience; and patience, experience; and experience, hope (Romans 5:3, 4).

The first week had been the toughest. Perry had paced back and forth past the refrigerator a thousand times. His hunger was so intense that it made him feel ill. He stuck with it a week, but he didn't lose much weight. He decided that he would diet at least one more week. Then it happened. A few pounds came off. Perry felt better. He felt more hopeful. The longer he dieted, the easier it got; especially when he could see some results.

Dieting is tough. It takes a lot of patience to wait for the first few results, but when they finally come, they offer us the hope we need to stick with it.

Today's thought: God gives us hope in order to cope!

July 6

And let us not be weary in well doing: for in due season we shall reap, if we faint not (Galatians 6:9).

Janet was tired of dieting. She had been at it for almost six months. She looked better, and knew that she was doing the right thing. Taking the pounds off had been hard, but sometimes Janet felt that keeping them off was even harder. Thin people didn't understand that dieting wasn't just something to do to lose weight. For a person with weight problems, it had to be a way of life.

God knows that dieting is hard. He knows dieting can be a bore. More than that, He knows we need help to diet. Rely on God. He won't let you down.

Today's thought: I will take dieting one day at a time, one pound at a time!

July 7

But without faith it is impossible to please Him: for he that cometh to God must believe that he is, and that he is a rewarder of them that diligently seek him (Hebrews 11:6).

Tim always said that God really didn't help him much. The trouble was, Tim never did much for God, either. He rarely prayed, hardly went to church, and didn't even own a Bible. When someone suggested that Tim might go on a diet, he said dieting didn't do any good. Tim pursued a diet about as apathetically as he pursued God.

We will never succeed in anything unless we dedicate ourselves — body, mind, and soul — to achieving our goal. A deep and driving faith can be the perfect model for our diets. If we will strive to lose weight as much as we strive after God, He will bless our effort.

Today's thought: I'm giving everything I've got to losing weight!

July 8

Behold, we count them happy which endure. Ye have heard of the patience of Job, and have seen the end of the Lord; that the Lord is very pitiful, and of tender mercy (James 5:11).

Gretchen wanted the job so badly. The doctor had told her she had to lose twenty pounds in order to pass the physical. Tina and Ann also had to lose weight to join the company. After a couple of weeks, Tina gave up. One week later, Ann folded, too. They both told Gretchen she was wasting her time. Gretchen didn't care. She held on, got her position, and never once regretted all she had to do to get it. She thanked the Lord that she had the strength to hold on when her friends had given up. Without His help, she never would have made it.

Today's thought: Job lost everything, and God blessed him greatly for what he suffered. If Job can endure, so can I!

July 9

Wherefore the rather, brethren, give diligence to make your calling and election sure: for if ye do these things, ye shall never fail (2 Peter 1:10).

Beverly never let her Bible get very far away from her. At the first tiny pang of hunger, she grabbed it and immersed herself in the gospels. Feeding on the word of God was much better for her than feeding her face, and it always took her mind off her hunger. God wouldn't let her fall. He gave her strength and commitment when she needed it the most. Her diet had helped make her a much stronger person, spiritually. She had seen God's power to help her lose weight, and it had given her even more confidence in His power to do other things. Beverly knew that her diligence and perseverance came from God and nowhere else.

Today's thought: I'm keeping God between me and the refrigerator!

July 10

For I reckon that the sufferings of this present time are not worthy to be compared with the glory which shall be revealed to us (Romans 8:18).

Jimmy was fascinated by the cocoon. He had watched the caterpillar work on its new home for hours. Everyday he came in to look at the cocoon. When the monarch butterfly finally emerged, Jimmy was delighted.

God works some amazing miracles in nature. It shouldn't be so hard to believe that He will work such miracles in the lives of His people. Losing weight might not seem like a miracle, but for those who struggle with their weight, it often feels as if only a miracle will suffice. If God can transform a caterpillar into a beautiful butterfly, He certainly can help us when all we want is to lose weight.

Today's thought: I am one of God's miracles, and He will help me be my best!

July 11

But as God hath distributed to every man, as the Lord hath called every one, so let him walk . . . (1 Corinthians 7:17).

Karen got so angry. Her friend Angie had started her diet at the same time Karen began. They had shopped together, eaten together, exercised together, but Angie had lost seven pounds more. It wasn't fair. What was the use of dieting when she couldn't lose weight as fast as her friend? She put forth the same effort, but got less reward.

God has made each of His children differently. No two are exactly alike. We are called by God to do our best with what we are given. We may not have the same results on our diet that others have on theirs, but that's okay. God will bless us for what we do, and that's what really counts.

Today's thought: God will help me lose my weight without losing my mind!

July 12

For do I now persuade men, or God? or do I seek to please men? for if I yet please men, I should not be the servant of Christ (Galatians 1:10).

Granny wanted Ellen to lose weight. She used to offer her bribes all the time, to encourage her. The problem was, no matter how much weight Ellen lost, her grandmother wanted her to lose more. There was just no pleasing her. Instead of helping Ellen lose weight, Granny just made her more frustrated and discouraged. It wasn't until Ellen decided she wanted to lose weight for herself that it really worked for her. She prayed for God's help, and He delivered. Doing it for Granny wasn't enough, doing it for God and herself made it all worthwhile.

Today's thought: The more I care, the less I weigh!

July 13

For we are his workmanship, created in Christ Jesus unto good works, which God hath before ordained that we should walk in them (Ephesians 2:10).

Randy couldn't believe how tough Bob's dad was on Bob. What was even more amazing was that Bob didn't seem to mind. Randy would have gone crazy if his own father demanded so much from him. Bob told him that his father was really a wonderful person and that he only wanted him to be the best person he could possibly be. Randy found it hard to believe, but one thing he did know: He sure wished he had as close a relationship with his own father as Bob had with his.

Our heavenly Father expects a lot from us. He wants us to be everything we can be. Though He's tough on us at times, He will always stand beside us to help us when we try to improve.

Today's thought: When we aren't tough enough on ourselves, God will be as tough as we need Him to be!

July 14

Being confident of this very thing, that he which hath begun a good work in you will perform it until the day of Jesus Christ (Philippians 1:6).

Ron was one of the best contractors in the business. Every job he'd ever started, he'd completed to the client's satisfaction. He never left anything undone. His reputation was beyond reproach.

No one ever had to worry when they had Ron working for them.

When we rely on God to help us with our dieting, we can rest assured that He will stick with us throughout the entire process. God does not give up. When he begins a job, He finishes it. We can have complete confidence in God. He will help us realize our goal.

Today's thought: With God's help, I can see this thing through to the end!

July 15

Whereunto I also labour, striving according to his working, which worketh in me mightily (Colossians 1:29).

Gail couldn't believe how much her life was changing. All through college, Gail hadn't even set foot in a church. The only social situation she had been comfortable in was where food was involved. College had been lonely and unfulfilling, not to mention fattening. Just recently she had attended church with her new neighbor, and it was like coming home. She felt comfortable and accepted. Her newfound relationship with Jesus Christ gave her a different perspective on her life. She suddenly found a deep concern for her appearance and health. As God became more and more a part of her life, Gail vowed to become the best person she could possibly be.

Today's thought: God's might is greater than my appetite!

July 16

For verily, when we were with you, we told you before that we should suffer tribulation; even as it came to pass, and ye know (1 Thessalonians 3:4).

Why don't diets get any easier? Chocolate cake is just as tempting a month or two after you start dieting as it is the day after you start. Time doesn't heal the cravings that go along with diets. There is suffering in dieting. For that reason, a good attitude and strong state of mind are essential for a productive, long-lasting diet. God gives us strength of character and determination. There is no tribulation, even dieting, that God can't get us through. Diets may not ever get easy, but they do get manageable when we add God's strength and perseverance to our own.

Today's thought: What seems impossible, God makes possible!

July 17

And if a man also strive for masteries, yet is he not crowned, except he strive lawfully (2 Timothy 2:5).

Susan lay looking up at the ceiling in her hospital room. She couldn't believe everything had turned out as it did. Jill had promised the pills were safe and that she would lose weight fast. All the pills had done were to make her violently ill and land her in the hospital.

Shortcuts are not the answer. God has given us willpower and a miraculous body that repairs itself if we give it the chance. Dieting doesn't require chemicals or radical exercising. Dieting requires mastery over our base desires and our selfish natures. Rely on God. We need nothing else.

Today's thought: God can do more to help me than anything else I could find!

July 18

If others be partakers of this power over you, are not we rather? Nevertheless we have not used this power; but suffer all things, lest we should hinder the gospel of Christ (1 Corinthians 9:12).

Betty got so annoyed with Sarah. Sarah had lost so much weight, but whenever anyone asked her how she did it, she told them she couldn't have done it without God's help. That got old really fast. Why didn't she just take credit and let it go at that? Everything had to be a big spiritual production for Sarah!

It's hard for some people to actually realize the power that Christians find in Jesus Christ. They can't understand our gratitude and thankfulness. We are partakers in a great and wonderful power, and it is right for us to acknowledge the source of that power. Christ saves lives, and He liberates us from things like obesity that threaten to make life less than it was meant to be.

Today's thought: I will give thanks to God for His help in my diet!

July 19

I have fought a good fight, I have finished my course, I have kept the faith (2 Timothy 4:7).

Bonnie took a good long look in the mirror. Amazing. She never thought she'd look this good again in her life. All the pain and torture and sacrifice was well worth it. She still couldn't believe it.

She had dreamed of the day she would feel really good about her dieting, and that day had arrived. What a great feeling!

If we will persevere, the day of triumph will indeed come. Like Paul, we need to fight the good fight, keep the faith, and complete the course. God promises to reward those who remain steadfast. Hold on to your dream and God will bless you richly.

Today's thought: I am closer to my goal with each passing day!

July 20

I press toward the mark for the prize of the high calling of God in Christ Jesus (Philippians 3:14).

Stan lived to please people. He served his church, his job, and his family with total devotion. He was continually asking what he could do for others. There was nothing Stan would not do in order to please someone else. Stan had never worried about his weight until one Sunday when the pastor read that his body was the Lord's temple. From that day forward, Stan worked to make it a fit and healthy temple. Not only was God pleased at Stan's desire to improve himself, but He was also pleased by the example Stan set for others.

Today's thought: I can actually glorify God just by losing weight!

July 21

Continue in prayer, and watch in the same with thanksgiving (Colossians 4:2).

Jane couldn't believe how much harder it was to diet now that Dottie had moved away. The strength and support of having someone to diet with had been immense. Just having someone to talk to had helped a lot. Now there was no one close by to say, "No!" The only thing that was saving Jane was her reliance on God. Whenever she found herself tempted and wishing for Dottie's support, she closed her eyes and talked to God. His presence assured Jane, and she was able to withstand temptation. It was good to have God as close as a prayer. For that she was eternally grateful.

Today's thought: Help in time of temptation is just one prayer away!

July 22

Have we not power to eat and to drink? (1 Corinthians 9:4)

Kevin blamed the diets. Kevin blamed his friends. Kevin blamed a bad childhood, glands, communists, and a government plot. Kevin blamed everyone but Kevin. Kevin tried and Kevin failed, but he never learned to take responsibility for his obesity.

We can never hope to get anywhere unless we are willing to take ownership of our own problems. God has given us freedom of choice. We have the ability to abuse that privilege if we so desire. It is our choice, however, and we control our own destiny. Dieting is nothing more than learning to tame a freedom that has degenerated into gluttony. God will help us tame that beast.

Today's thought: I'm in control of my life; my stomach isn't.

July 23

. . . we ourselves glory in you in the churches of God for your patience and faith in all your persecutions and tribulations that ye endure (2 Thessalonians 1:4).

Ed was on a severely restricted diet by order of his doctor. There were more foods he couldn't have than there were that he could. Almost everyone felt sorry for him, because they knew how much Ed loved his food. The only person who didn't seem to feel sorry for Ed was Ed. He accepted his fate with a smile and a shrug. His ability to adjust was a testimony to his faith and character. Many people found comfort in Ed's ability to take his diet in stride. His perseverance showed many people that it could be done. Through something so simple, God managed to touch the lives of many.

Today's thought: My diet is only as big a deal as I make it!

July 24

I will instruct thee and teach thee in the way which thou shalt go: I will guide thee with mine eye (Psalms 32:8).

Terry had been a savior. It was so nice to find someone who had gone through a long, hard diet before. God had really brought them together. At the time Lisa needed someone most, Terry had miraculously showed up. Lisa wondered whether Terry wasn't an angel in disguise. She had been such a great help.

God often answers our prayers through the people He sends into our lives at key times. It is good to seek out the support of others who can relate to what we're going through. Pray that God will lead you to such people, so they might accompany you through the tough times.

Today's thought: Help me remember that I'm not alone!

July 25

This I say then, Walk in the Spirit, and ye shall not fulfil the lust of the flesh (Galatians 5:16).

Dan made a resolution to use his breakfast and lunch times for prayer and reflection. He would eat something light, then spend the rest of the time in quiet time with God. It got him through some really tough periods of hunger and temptation. Refreshed by the time with God, Dan then no longer felt the desire to stuff himself. God strengthened him, gave him courage, and filled him with resistance enough to persevere.

God will fill the emptiness we feel in our bellies. He will fill us with His own Holy Spirit and lead us away from temptation. Rely on God. His strength is offered to all who will but receive it.

Today's thought: I would rather be spirit filled instead of calorie filled!

July 26

For I am in a strait betwixt two, having a desire to depart, and to be with Christ; which is far better: Nevertheless to abide in the flesh is more needful for you (Philippians 1:23, 24).

Paul questioned why God had put him on earth in the first place. Being fat seemed like unnecessary torture. The diets were killers, and they didn't seem to do any good, anyway. What was the use of trying and failing over and over again? Better to never have been born.

Despair and frustration are a part of dieting. Often it seems so hopeless. Still, God has given us life as a gift. We prepare ourselves in this life for eternal life in God's presence. Now is the time we need to learn self-discipline and control. Now is the time to strive to be everything we are meant to be. Our life in the flesh is necessary, and it is up to us to make sure we take proper care of ourselves.

Today's thought: I'll try my hardest to lose weight today, because I may not get another chance!

July 27

That if thou shalt confess with thy mouth the Lord Jesus, and shalt believe in thine heart that God hath raised him from the dead, thou shalt be saved (Romans 10:9).

Why do so many people believe that God has absolute power over life and death but doubt whether He can do anything to help them transform a small part of their own lives? Why should a few pounds of flesh be a more insurmountable obstacle than a mountain or a stone that sealed a tomb? True faith reminds us that our Lord is the Lord of the impossible. He enables us to rise above our limitations through the power of the Holy Spirit. Our God must be the Lord of the diet, too. The Lord who resurrected Jesus the Christ on Easter morning will faithfully resurrect us from a tomb of obesity and flesh. Trust in God's power, for by it we are saved.

Today's thought: I need Jesus to save me from me!

July 28

The husbandman that laboureth must be first partaker of the fruits (2 Timothy 2:6).

Wendy thought she was dieting for her husband and family. She kept telling herself she was doing it for them, anyway. As the pounds melted away, however, Wendy realized something very important. No matter who she said she was doing it for, she came out the big winner. She looked better, she felt better, and she loved every minute of it. She knew she was doing something really right. She put forth a lot of sweat and tears, and she was reaping the big benefits. Not only was she dieting for her family, but she was doing it for herself, and that was a good thing. She was worth it.

Today's thought: My diet is a really great decision on my part!

July 29

I therefore, the prisoner of the Lord, beseech you that ye walk worthy of the vocation wherewith ye are called (Ephesians 4:1).

Rodney let himself go completely. His friends were uncomfortable when he was around. He ate constantly, and he seemed to grow larger by the day. No one knew how to talk to him about it, so they let it slide. Finally, Barb took him aside and asked him why he was destroying himself. She told him that people were losing their respect for him and couldn't understand it. In anger, Rodney told Barb it was none of her business and stormed off.

As Christians, it is other people's business when we follow paths that are not worthy of Jesus Christ. He has called us to be living examples of Himself. To be less than that is a sin. Let us try to live life in a body fit for Christ.

Today's thought: Do people see Christ when they look at me?

July 30

And whatsoever ye do, do it heartily, as to the Lord, and not unto men (Colossians 3:23).

Alice was right: Doug had been doing his diet halfway. His heart hadn't really been in it, and Alice asked him why he was even doing it at all. Now, he felt he was ready. Alice had offered the challenge, and he aimed to take her up on it. No more halfway measures: he was going to throw all his energy and commitment into losing some weight.

God wants us to mean what we say. Our yes must mean yes, and our no must mean no. Whatever we choose to do, we ought to do it fully, for God wants children with commitment and resolve, not indecision and insincerity.

Today's thought: My diet is an all-or-nothing proposition!

July 31

As the whirlwind passeth, so is the wicked no more: but the righteous is an everlasting foundation (Proverbs 10:25).

When the group began, there were sixteen people involved. They all made a contract to lose twenty pounds by spring. Spring was less than two weeks away, and the group was down to seven members. As Jean walked along the sidewalk toward the building where her group met, she noticed some small saplings bending in the stiff March breeze. Some had broken off, but a few determined little plants held on for dear life. "I'm like that," Jean thought. "Most of the others have given up, but I'm going to hang in there, no matter how stiff the challenge." Perseverance is a huge part of a successful diet. Continually ask God for commitment to your cause. He is good to give it.

Today's thought: I'm determined to make it, no matter what!

AUGUST
Comfort

When we attempt anything that is difficult and painful, we need comfort in order to survive the ordeal. God has placed within us a need to be comforted, but also a need to comfort. We can find comfort in the fact that God is with us in our diet, millions of other people are with us in spirit in our diet, and we usually have friends to turn to as we diet. All these avenues of comfort are vital as we try to change our lives by losing weight. As we find comfort through the tough times in our diets, we also find strength and courage. God blesses us with everything we need, if we only turn to Him and include Him in our weight-loss programs. There is no greater source of comfort than the Lord. We can turn to Him in our times of greatest need, and He will soothe and comfort us every time.

August 1
I will not leave you comfortless: I will come to you (John 14:18).

Joan was such a great friend. Almost every day she would stop by to see how things were going. Joan had been there herself. She had battled her weight for years. It was comforting to have someone around who had made it. Joan looked great. Just knowing it could be done made the whole diet easier, somehow.

When we try to lose weight all by ourselves, the struggle is doubly difficult. We all need support in tough times. We can count on God's comfort when we diet. He has promised that He will never leave us comfortless. Believe in that promise. When our diets seem most futile, God will come to us.

Today's thought: With the help of friends, I can lose more pounds!

August 2
Come unto me, all ye that labour and are heavy laden, and I will give you rest (Matthew 11:28).

Sunday was "anything goes" day. Carol had decided that if she was good about sticking to her diet through the week, she would allow herself to splurge on Sunday. It made the diet so much more tolerable. Interestingly, she never really went overboard on Sunday. She ate something she really liked, but she ate a moderate amount and found herself totally satisfied.

Whenever we attempt something difficult, we need to allow ourselves a respite. It is a good thing to take a break, even from a diet. It requires self-control, but it can help us keep a healthy perspective on why we diet in the first place. Once we have rested from our fast, we can return to it renewed.

Today's thought: I am tired of being heavy ladened physically!

August 3

Peace I leave with you, my peace I give unto you: not as the world giveth, give I unto you. Let not your heart be troubled, neither let it be afraid (John 14:27).

Bill felt it was a no-win situation. If he dieted, he felt lousy because he was hungry all the time. If he broke his diet, he felt guilty. It was hard to tell which was worse, the hunger or the guilt. He wanted to trim down, but he loved to eat. He never knew that he'd suffer through so much turmoil just trying to lose weight.

Diets can really stir us up. They make us feel physically and emotionally strained. During periods of dieting, we need to find peace of mind and heart. Ask God for that peace. He promises to deliver it to those who ask Him for it. When we need it most, God gladly gives it.

Today's thought: Better to have peace of mind than a piece of cake!

August 4

For it is God which worketh in you both to will and to do of his good pleasure (Philippians 2:13).

Stephanie got fantastic grades in algebra. All her friends were jealous of her abilities in class. Stephanie always smiled to herself. None of her friends realized that her father was a scientist who used algebra all the time. He tutored her every evening and helped her understand the problems that gave her friends such fits.

There are times when we need special help. Without it we struggle twice as hard as we really need to. God offers to help us through our diets. Allow God to work within you as you diet, and you'll be surprised how much easier it is.

Today's thought: When the fat won't go away, take a moment then to pray!

August 5

He shall feed his flock like a shepherd: he shall gather the lambs with his arm, and carry them in his bosom, and shall gently lead those that are with young (Isaiah 40:11).

Mary blew it. She had been doing so well, then she gave in completely. In a week she gained back what had taken her a month to lose. Depressed, she called her mother for comfort. Mom was always good at that. If anyone could get her back on the right track, it was her mother. She could always trust her mother to give her sound, loving advice.

God is like that. We can trust that He will guide us along good paths. When we need someone to comfort us without condemnation, God is always there for us. He will gather us to Himself and make us ready to go on.

Today's thought: I may be weak, but I'm strong enough to call on God's help!

August 6

Though I walk in the midst of trouble, thou wilt revive me: thou shalt stretch forth thine hand against the wrath of mine enemies, and thy right hand shall save me (Psalms 138:7).

It was war! Greg looked at the bag of cookies on the table in front of him, and they almost made him cry. Why couldn't he just ignore them? It was as if they had some kind of magical spell over him. As long as there were cookies nearby, Greg felt he had to eat them. Closing his eyes didn't help. Neither did putting them in the cabinet; he still knew they were there. He was determined to resist their pull, but was he really strong enough?

When the temptations get to be too much, we need to call upon the Lord. In the midst of our stiffest challenges, He will truly save us.

Today's thought: I need God to save me from myself!

August 7

For the Lord shall be thy confidence, and shall keep thy foot from being taken (Proverbs 3:26).

Norm felt drowsy, but he didn't want to stop. He only had a few miles to go, to get home. Home. He began thinking about how nice it would be to get there and fall into a comfortable bed. Before he knew it, he was dropping off to sleep. He came to with a jolt as his fender scraped along the guardrail at the side of the road. Thank God for the guardrail. Without it, Norm didn't know where he'd be.

We need guardrails. They keep us from pitching off into nothingness; past the point of no return. God can be our guardrail, keeping us from indulging our appetites past reasonable limitations. Truly, He keeps us from falling.

Today's thought: Food is a trap I'd rather not fall into!

August 8
And the light shineth in darkness; and the darkness compre-
hended it not (John 1:5).

Rusty scared herself. She walked past the mirror in the dim light
of dusk and thought there was a stranger in the house. How had
she gotten so big? Who was she kidding? She kept telling herself
that she wasn't that big, but it was so bad she didn't recognize
herself in the mirror. It was like a revelation: a bright light shining
through the darkness. She had to do something about her weight.
Determined, she set out to lose the weight she had gained, and
with God's help, she was able to do just that.

Today's thought: I want to find out just how good I can look!

August 9
When Jesus had lifted up himself, and saw none but the
woman, he said unto her, Woman, where are those thine ac-
cusers? hath no man condemned thee? She said, No man, Lord.
And Jesus said unto her, Neither do I condemn thee: go, and sin
no more (John 8:10, 11).

The doctor was going to kill her. Kate had been told to lose thirty
pounds over six months. For awhile she had done really well. She
took off twenty in the first three months, but lately she had gained
again, for a net loss of only about twelve pounds. Kate was
astonished when the doctor merely told her to try harder.
Christ, like the doctor, offers us no condemnation. He wants us
to lose weight for our own sakes, not for His. He wants to help us,
not hurt us. Take comfort in the acceptance of Jesus Christ.

Today's thought: Even when I give in, I'm still a good person.

August 10
For there is no respect of persons with God (Romans 2:11).

Andrea was furious. She hadn't wanted to go on the hike in the
first place, and now she was falling farther and farther behind. No
one would give her time to catch up. Some of them were even
laughing at her. It wasn't her fault she wasn't in good physical
condition. She had to carry around a lot more weight than they
did. It just wasn't fair.
In this life, we don't get a lot of breaks. Just because we're overweight doesn't mean we deserve special treatment. God doesn't
give preferential treatment. He wants all of His children to be the
best they can possibly be. He expects us all to do our best.

Today's thought: I am trying my best to please God!

August 11
And he said to the woman, Thy faith hath saved thee; go in peace (Luke 7:50).

God will help us as we diet, but the weight of the responsibility still lies with us. We have to really want to lose weight. God will not do it for us. Faith is the key to unlocking God's power in our lives. When we put our faith in God, He is able to lead us in new ways. He fills us with strength, courage, purpose, and the will to succeed. God has already placed those qualities in each one of us. Faith is our way of allowing God to show us how to use what we've already got. Let us remain open to God so we can succeed in losing the weight that doesn't need to be there.

Today's thought: God has given me everything I need to fight fat!

August 12
But God, who is rich in mercy, for his great love wherewith he loved us, even when we were dead in sins, hath quickened us together with Christ, (by grace ye are saved) (Ephesians 2:4, 5).

It really isn't a matter of whether God loves us more if we're thin than He does if we're fat. God loves us the same, no matter what. He loves sinners as much as He loves saints. His greatest desire, though, is for His children to be everything they can be. He wants us to desire perfection. The gluttony and selfishness that lead to obesity are not qualities of perfection. God wants us to attempt to live our lives as Jesus lived His. Let us vow to walk in a newness of life, transformed by the power of the Holy Spirit, on the road to Christlike perfection.

Today's thought: God can make me better than I ever dreamed possible!

August 13
Comfort ye, comfort ye my people, saith your God (Isaiah 40:1).

Josh was feeling down and depressed. Nothing seemed to be working out for him. His job was a nightmare, his social life was even worse, and he was lonely. He sat alone and ate. His weight had skyrocketed. He wouldn't eat so much if he had someone to talk to. His main problem was that he just didn't have anything else to do.

Often, the most comforting thing we can hope for is someone to spend time with. Company gives us pleasure and takes our mind off eating. It is up to us to find people to spend time with when that is the only reason we sit and stuff ourselves. God sends us comfort in many ways. Seek the comfort of company.

Today's thought: I'm never so tempted to cheat as when I'm alone!

August 14

And let the peace of God rule in your hearts, to the which also ye are called in one body; and be ye thankful (Colossians 3:15).

Scott was cranky. He had been on a diet for two weeks, and it wasn't getting easier. Now his friends wanted to drag him off to some stupid prayer meeting at the church. Begrudgingly, Scott agreed to go. Before long, his mind was off of food and on to the message the pastor was delivering. Scott got caught up in praying for the needs of others, and he completely forgot about his own hunger. The time passed quickly, and Scott was surprised. His friends just smiled and told Scott that there was a lesson there for him somewhere.

When we turn our attention from ourselves to others, great things can happen.

Today's thought: I want to care for others as much as I care about myself!

August 15

And I heard a great voice out of heaven saying, Behold, the tabernacle of God is with men, and he will dwell with them, and they shall be his people, and God himself shall be with them, and be their God (Revelation 21:3).

Cathy decided to make a contract with God rather than a promise to herself. She vowed that she would lose weight for Him, not for any vain or selfish reason she could come up with. Somehow it was easier to do for God than it had been for herself. The pounds melted much quicker. Cathy continued her diet with regular prayer and recommitment to the promise she made to God. Before long, Kathy had lost all the weight she set out to lose.

Our promises to God are very important. Often we can do for Him what we fail at for ourselves. God has promised to help us whenever we need Him. He will help us lose weight.

Today's thought: My diet is more than a wish; it is a promise to God.

August 16

Wherefore comfort yourselves together, and edify one another, even as also ye do (1 Thessalonians 5:11).

Joining the group was the best move she ever made. Fay had struggled alone through a dozen diets with no real success. Then she saw the notice on the church bulletin board about the group that dieted and exercised together. She was a little hesitant at first, but finally she decided to give it a try. What a difference it made! Dieting with a group was much better than dieting alone. Fay felt that God had really led her to this group. She gained so much strength from her new friends, and she was amazed at how much she was able to help others.

Today's thought: A diet for two is easier to do!

August 17

Behold, he that keepeth Israel shall neither slumber nor sleep. The Lord is thy keeper: the Lord is thy shade upon thy right hand (Psalms 121:4, 5).

The Hebrew people had great confidence in God. They believed His promises to them, and they lived their lives accordingly. No matter how difficult their situation got, the children of Israel held onto their faith. Through that faith, they were able to do amazing things.

The God of Abraham and Isaac is also the God of Jesus Christ. If we will put our faith in Him, He will enable us to do amazing things. He will allow us to lose the weight we need to lose, and He will comfort us when our diets get particularly tough. Trust in the Lord. He is watching over you.

Today's thought: I'd better watch what I eat as closely as God watches me!

August 18

Are not two sparrows sold for a farthing? and one of them shall not fall on the ground without your Father. Fear ye not therefore, ye are of more value than many sparrows (Matthew 10:29, 31).

Jeff was suspicious. He couldn't figure out why his friends were trying to be so helpful with his diet. What could they possibly get out of it? Whenever he was with them, they avoided talking about food, and they ate salads and cottage cheese instead of normal food. They wouldn't even have dessert. It made Jeff feel a little awkward and guilty. He couldn't believe his friends would go to so much trouble to help him out.

Some people wonder whether or not God really cares about their diet problems. The fact is, He cares about everything that is important to us. Take comfort in the fact that God cares deeply, and He will do everything He can to help you.

Today's thought: God thinks I'm great, with or without weight!

August 19

For God sent not his Son into the world to condemn the world; but that the world through him might be saved (John 3:17).

Guilt. Every time Liz slipped, she felt guilty. Her husband gave her such disapproving looks. She wanted to stick to her diet, but it was hard. Then, when people made her feel guilty, she got depressed, which only made her want to eat more. The more she ate, the guiltier she felt; the guiltier she felt, the more she ate. It was a vicious cycle. She wished people would be more understanding. She honestly believed that would make all the difference.

We don't need pressure put on us by those who condemn us for not being perfect. That's why God is the perfect diet mate. He supports without condemning, and He loves us even when we fail.

Today's thought: I can do wonderful things with God's support!

August 20

And Jesus answered and said unto her, Martha, Martha, thou art careful and troubled about many things: but one thing is needful: and Mary hath chosen that good part, which shall not be taken away from her (Luke 10:41, 42).

Angie brought home a new diet book each week. She had a closet full of exercisers guaranteed to take off pounds and inches. She had a cabinet full of pills, powders, and liquids bearing promises of miraculous weight loss. Cindy just shook her head. Why go to all the trouble? Losing weight wasn't going to come from anywhere except from inside the person who wanted to lose it. Desire was the main ingredient. It was too easy to get caught up in fads and fancy claims. A quiet determination to lose weight was what was really important. Angie lost a few pounds, while Cindy lost many.

Today's thought: It's hard to lose weight when you have a fat head!

August 21

If a man therefore purge himself from these, he shall be a vessel unto honour, sanctified, and meet for the master's use, and prepared unto every good work (2 Timothy 2:21).

Gary couldn't believe what he was hearing. He hadn't been selected for the mission because he was just a few pounds overweight. Harrison was trimmer, but that didn't mean he was any better as a pilot. How could they turn him down because of a few pounds.

Often being fit is determined by how trim and slim we are. It may not be fair, but it shows the value that is put on keeping in shape. God wants us to be in shape so we can enjoy this life we have been given to the fullest. He intends that we should always be ready to experience all that life has to offer. We can only do that when we take proper care of ourselves.

Today's thought: I am making myself fit for life!

August 22

But after that the kindness and love of God our Saviour toward man appeared, not by works of righteousness which we have done, but according to his mercy he saved us, by the washing of regeneration, and renewing of the Holy Ghost (Titus 3:4, 5).

It was a miraculous metamorphosis. Darleen had lost one hundred pounds. Though everyone encouraged her as much as possible, no one really believed she could do it. The proof was before their eyes: Darleen looked great. Someone asked her how she had done it, and she told them that a crisis in her life had made her realize she didn't just need to lose weight, she needed to be saved from her own body. She fell in her kitchen and had not been able to get up again. Through her pain and frustration, she believed she was being taught a valuable lesson. She thanked God that He had gotten through to her before it was too late.

Today's thought: Save me from being a prisoner to obesity!

August 23

Who shall separate us from the love of Christ! shall tribulation, or distress, or persecution, or famine, or nakedness, or peril, or sword? Nay, in all these things we are more than conquereors through him that loved us (Romans 8:35, 37).

Christ makes us conquerors. He offers us unimaginable power through the Holy Spirit. Nothing can separate us from that love and power. That power enabled Jesus Christ to conquer death. It allowed the Apostle Paul to conquer his afflictions. It allowed Peter to overcome his doubts and fears. If the Holy Spirit could do that for those great men, then why shouldn't we be able to believe that the Spirit will help us lose weight? Indeed, we can even conquer obesity through the divine power of God. Nothing can stop us from achieving our goal, because the power of God is with us.

Today's thought: I will burn up calories in the fire of the Holy Spirit!

August 24

For we have great joy and consolation in thy love, because the bowels of the saints are refreshed by thee, brother (Philemon 1:7).

Phil had a lousy self-image. He felt unwanted and unloved. He looked at himself in the mirror and saw an enormous slob. No one could love that. Dieting didn't even make sense. It was useless. Nothing would ever change.

Poor Phil honestly believed he was unloved. He had no reason to change because he saw no hope for his future. How sad that Phil didn't know the love of God. We can proceed with our diets knowing that we are loved and that we are lovable. Just knowing that makes it all worthwhile. We draw strength from the comfort that comes from being loved. That strength ensures that we can lose the weight we want to lose.

Today's thought: Special people can do anything they set their mind to, and I am a special person!

August 25

Judge not, and ye shall not be judged: condemn not, and ye shall not be condemned: forgive, and ye shall be forgiven (Luke 6:37).

Kelly was unbearable. She had lost thirty pounds with relative ease, so she ridiculed anyone who couldn't do it as easily as she had. Kelly wasn't being fair. Every person is different. It didn't mean that others weren't as committed or as dedicated as Kelly had been. It was frustrating to try so hard and then have Kelly make fun of you for it. Why couldn't she have a little compassion? After all, she had been obese once!

After losing weight, we should be more compassionate than anyone else. It is important to remember how hard losing weight really is. We have a wonderful opportunity to help others when we keep in mind what we've had to come through.

Today's thought: I hope I can lose my weight without losing my sensitivity toward others!

August 26

And the Lord shall deliver me from every evil work, and will preserve me unto his heavenly kingdom: to whom be glory for ever and ever. Amen (2 Timothy 4:18).

Wes looked at the sign on the refrigerator door: God is watching! What a thought! Everything he did was under God's watchful eye. A slight groan escaped his lips as he thought of the times he'd cheated through the week. He hoped it was worth it. Actually, Wes kind of liked the sign. It make him think, and once he got to thinking, his diet wasn't so bad. God had helped him avoid a lot of unnecessary snacks. There were worse things to have happen to you than to have God watching every move you made. Wes felt pretty confident. With God's help, he was really going to make it through this thing!

Today's thought: God's steering me clear of the fat traps!

August 27
For he is our peace, who hath made both one, and hath broken down the middle wall of partition between us; having abolished in his flesh the enmity, even the law of commandments contained in ordinances; for to make in himself of twain one new man, so making peace (Ephesians 2:14, 15).

As wrong as it was, Rachel had to admit that being thin helped her fit in. She really wasn't a different person now that she was thin, but people sure treated her that way. It was unbelievable that people were so biased against those who were fat. Rachel sighed a prayer of thankfulness to God that He had helped her lose weight. It was hard, being on the outside. Nobody likes being ostracized. She also prayed that God might make people see how unfair it was to judge others based on their appearance. If God could help Rachel lose weight, perhaps He could change the bigotry of some concerning obesity.

Today's thought: Fat or skinny, I'm the same person inside!

August 28
And ye shall be my people, and I will be your God (Jeremiah 30:22).

The covenant that God made was quite simple: He would be God to a group of people who would accept Him and honor Him. God's promises are always simple and straightforward. There are never strings attached. God will do everything He can to help us deal with this life. He wants to see His children happy and fulfilled. That is why He will help us when we need His comforting strength. Alone, we just don't have what it takes to make it. With God, however, there is no force on earth great enough to keep us from our goal. Remember God, and truly He will remember you in time of need.

Today's thought: My willpower comes from the strongest power source around!

August 29
That he would grant you, according to the riches of his glory, to be strengthened with might by his Spirit in the inner man (Ephesians 3:16).

Herm couldn't figure out why he wasn't losing weight. He knew he wasn't eating as much as he had before he retired. When he was on the road, he ate like a horse. Now that he was home around the house all the time, he ate a lot less. Something definitely wasn't right.

Losing weight requires much more than just changing our eating habits. We need to change our whole outlook on things. Sometimes we need to cut back on food while increasing the amount of exercise we get. Other times we need to give up certain foods altogether. We need to evaluate deep inside how we live out our lives, and make adjustments necessary to succeed in losing weight.

Today's thought: Dieting doesn't happen on its own. It takes a conscious effort!

August 30

Now our Lord Jesus Christ himself, and God, even our Father, which hath loved us, and hath given us everlasting consolation and good hope through grace, comfort your hearts, and stablish you in every good word and work (2 Thessalonians 2:16, 17).

Another diet. Carla had tried so many times, and she had never come close to succeeding. She wasn't even sure why she was trying again. She knew it would be good for her to lose weight, but she felt beaten before she even began. What would make this time any different from the rest?

What makes one attempt different from others is this: confidence. We really have to believe that we can do it. It should help us immensely to know that God believes in us. He knows us better than we know ourselves, and He has equipped us with everything we need to succeed. All we have to do is learn to believe.

Today's thought: What I lack in confidence. I make up for with faith!

August 31

Now the Lord of peace himself give you peace always by all means. The Lord be with you all (2 Thessalonians 3:16).

Ted felt the material rip the moment he bent over. Funny, that never happened a few years ago. Either his clothes were all shrinking or he was filling out a bit. There was just one thing to do about it: He was going to have to lose a few pounds. He'd done it before; he could do it again. A little willpower, a little patience, and a few prayers for strength. Ted was a man who knew his God and believed He would help out. He had never doubted Him, and God had never let him down. It was nice to feel so confident about something. Dieting was easy when you were positive that God would help you work things out.

Today's thought: I'm going to wear clothes I haven't fit into in years!

SEPTEMBER
Doubt

Whenever we involve ourselves in a process that takes time, it is only natural to move through periods of doubt. Doubt is not necessarily a bad thing. It can help us reassess our desires and motives. We ask ourselves why we are doing what we do. People diet for all different reasons, some of them good, some of them not so good. When the pounds don't fall quite as fast as we think they should, it causes us to feel frustrated and hopeless. Doubt sets in. If we are to fight the negative effects of doubt, we will definitely need help. We can turn to friends for help when the doubts mount up, but more importantly, we can turn to God, who knows what is on our heart before we even speak to Him. He will be true to strengthen and encourage us. In the light of Christ, even our darkest doubts are dispelled. Open your heart to the light of Christ and experience the joy as your doubts fade into nothingness.

September 1
Not that we are sufficient of ourselves to think any thing as of ourselves; but our sufficiency is of God (2 Corinthians 3:5).

Muriel knew she couldn't do it alone. She wasn't strong enough. Her friend Ann told her that one of her strengths was realizing she was weak. Too many of her friends tackled diets on their own and failed miserably. Well, Muriel wasn't going to make the same mistake. She wanted help from the outset.

If we realize our weaknesses and limitations, then we are better able to cope with them. God will help us be honest with ourselves, so we can work to turn our weaknesses into strengths. Pray to God for that insight.

Today's thought: What I *want* to eat and what I *need* to eat are two different things!

September 2
Fear thou not; for I am with thee: be not dismayed; for I am thy God: I will strengthen thee; yea, I will help thee; yea, I will uphold thee with the right hand of my righteousness (Isaiah 41:10).

Ben was afraid to even try a diet. He never had much luck with things that required a lot of willpower on his part. He caved in much too easily. If only someone else would make his decisions for him. He had never been overweight when he lived at home and had his mother around to tell him what to eat and what not to eat. Ben would be the first one to admit that he had no self-control.

Unfortunately, we all have to learn to discipline ourselves. God doesn't tell us what to do. He gives us complete freedom, but He will help us have the strength to make right decisions if we ask Him to. Include God, and He will make some wonderful things happen.

Today's thought: True power is the ability to say no!

September 3
For I am the Lord, I change not; therefore ye sons of Jacob are not consumed (Malachi 3:6).

God was such a big help when Gwen began her diet, but He didn't seem to care much anymore. Lately, Gwen's diet had become almost intolerable. She began to wonder if God knew what she was going through. She had prayed daily when she started her diet, and it had gotten so easy that she really didn't need to pray all the time. Then, it started getting harder. Why did God let that happen?

Poor Gwen never realized that God hadn't changed, but she had. She included God all the time at first, then she left Him out more and more. God will help us just as much as we allow Him to. Often we are our own, and God's, worst enemy when we take our lives out of God's hands and put them into our own.

Today's thought: God and I are dieting together!

September 4
Ask, and it shall be given you; seek, and ye shall find; knock, and it shall be opened unto you: For every one that asketh receiveth; and he that seeketh findeth; and to him that knocketh it shall be opened (Matthew 7:7, 8).

Barry never really believed that he'd lose the weight. That was probably his problem. His heart was never in it. Whenever he got the least bit discouraged, he'd immediately give up. His friends tried to offer support, but Barry always came up with excuses why he should give up his diet.

If we want to lose weight, we need to believe in ourselves. Self-doubt is a killer. If we lack faith in ourselves, then perhaps we can overcome it by the faith we have in God. God can fill us with a self-assurance that allows us to do almost anything we set our minds to. Push aside doubt. Be filled with the confidence of God.

Today's thought: With God's help, I'll knock off a few pounds!

September 5

The Lord is not slack concerning his promise, as some men count slackness; but is longsuffering to us-ward, not willing that any should perish, but that all should come to repentance (2 Peter 3:9).

Lois woke up from the strangest dream. She had died and gone to heaven, but when she got there, she couldn't get in. There was an extremely narrow hallway that everyone had to pass through before they could enter heaven. Try as she might, Lois couldn't get through the passageway because she was so large. Before, she had doubted that she could lose weight. Now, she found a new motivation. She believed God had broken through her excuses to tell her how important it was for her to lose. Never once did she believe that God would keep her out of heaven because of her weight, but she realized that her weight already kept her from enjoying life the way God intended it to be.

Today's thought: Life is great when you carry less weight!

September 6

Thou shalt make thy prayer unto him, and he shall hear thee, and thou shalt pay thy vows (Job 22:27).

Gary took time every morning to pray about his diet. Some days he awoke frustrated that he wasn't losing weight. Other days he awoke with cravings, afraid he wouldn't be able to withstand temptation. Still other mornings he just wanted to thank God that he'd come so far. God helped make the diet bearable. Every time Gary found himself feeling ready to give up, a quick prayer to God gave him the willpower to go on.

The power of God is a wonderful thing. We cannot comprehend how much God does for us when we call upon His name. Rest assured that God is with you in all you do . . . even your diet.

Today's thought: The more time you pray, the less you can weigh!

September 7

The righteous cry, and the Lord heareth, and delivereth them out of all their troubles (Psalms 34:17).

Pat lay crying in bed. It was so hard. It seems that for every three pounds she lost, she immediately gained two back. She really wanted to lose weight, but she felt so weak in the face of temptation. Wasn't there anything that could help her?

Pat fell asleep that night with a prayer on her lips. Strangely, she felt a wonderful peace the next morning. The battle was truly tough, but she was once more ready to face it. God didn't take away the struggle, but He was able to give Pat just what she needed to carry on. That is the wonder of our God.

Today's thought: I'll keep fighting fat until I'm fit!

September 8
And seek not ye what ye shall eat, or what ye shall drink, neither be ye of doubtful mind (Luke 12:29).

Clyde was so infuriating! Every time his wife suggested that he go on a diet, he came up with some excuse. Most of the time he just said that diets weren't healthy. He was afraid he would do more harm than good. Clyde knew it was just a dodge. He didn't want to lose weight, and he saw no reason why anyone should want to push him. That all changed when he landed in the hospital with a heart attack brought on because his body simply couldn't carry the weight Clyde contained. Clyde no longer questioned what was right. Instead of doubting the intelligence of dieting, he wondered why he had ever been so stupid as to resist it. Sometimes God needs to let us know through crisis what we will not hear normally.

Today's thought: If it's a choice between dieting or dying, I think I'll diet!

September 9
And the peace of God, which passeth all understanding, shall keep your hearts and minds through Christ Jesus (Philippians 4:7).

Jessica was doubtful at first. She really didn't believe Mindy when she said the church would be a big help during her diet. Mindy had taken her to see the pastor, and they had told him that they were dieting. She felt silly at first, but the pastor asked regularly how they were doing, and Jessica liked that. It made her feel that what she was doing was important and a good thing. Other members of the church mentioned how good they were looking. Before long, Jessica found that she enjoyed the dieting because she enjoyed the reactions of the church people and didn't want to let them down. Mindy was right: the church helped a lot.

Today's thought: Sharing the load of dieting makes the burden light!

September 10
For God hath not given us the spirit of fear; but of power, and of love, and of a sound mind (2 Timothy 1:7).

Brenda decided it was time to lose weight, and she did. Peggy struggled a little bit more, but she lost the pounds she wanted to, also. Tracy wondered why everyone else seemed to do so well, while she did so poorly. Maybe something was wrong with her! Maybe she couldn't lose weight. The more she thought about it, the more frightened she became.

Often our mind turns out to be our worst enemy when we try to diet. We can alarm ourselves needlessly. Everyone diets differently, and everyone receives different results. There is no place for fear and doubting in dieting. What we need is perseverance and faith that God will help us.

Today's thought: I have a very skinny spirit!

September 11
And being fully persuaded that, what he had promised, he was able also to perform (Romans 4:21).

Jesus Christ turned water to wine. He walked on the water and calmed the sea. He cured many diseases and cast out demons. He conquered death for His friend Lazarus and for Himself. He promises that He will be with us and that His power is ours as we try to be the people God created us to be. How, then, can we doubt that He will help us when we need to lose weight? Are not the pounds of our flesh within His scope of power? Cannot the chosen Son of God do such a small miracle in our lives as to give us the determination we need to conquer fat? This He can and will do, and much more, if we will but believe.

Today's thought: "More" brought about my distress; help me, Lord, to live by "less!"

September 12
Set your affection on things above, not on things on the earth (Colossians 3:2).

The smells from the cafeteria were more than Blanche could take. Not that the cafeteria food was anything to write home about, but when she was on a diet, almost anything smelled good! She grabbed her jacket and headed out the door. Immediately, the fresh fall air erased the cafeteria smells. The sky was a deep blue, and the white clouds lazily drifted by. The sun was out, the birds were singing, and everything was right with the world. Blanche spent her lunch hour just strolling through God's splendor. Before she knew it, her hunger had passed, and she was ready to tackle the afternoon. The glory of God had lifted her above her earthly passions, and she was grateful.

Today's thought: There's much more to life than lunch!

111

September 13

Thou wilt keep him in perfect peace, whose mind is stayed on thee: because he trusteth in thee (Isaiah 26:3).

Bud believed his doctor really did have his best interests in mind. Bud wouldn't have dieted if anyone else had told him he should but his doctor carried a little more weight. Bud kept to the diet because he felt it was the right thing to do. Trust was a big factor in making everything work.

Trust is a big factor in anything we try to do. Giants of the Christian faith were able to do such great things because they trusted that the Lord was with them. We, perhaps not giants of the faith, need to rest assured that we can trust God and that He will do everything He can to help us lose weight.

Today's thought: The only thing God will let down is my weight!

September 14

When thou liest down, thou shalt not be afraid: yea, thou shalt lie down, and thy sleep shall be sweet (Proverbs 3:24).

Janice remembered long, sleepless nights where she tossed and turned, feeling guilty that she had cheated on her diet or merely crying because she was so enormous. Thank God those nights were long gone. Being fat was not just a physical trauma, but an emotional and mental one, as well. She never realized how much her peace of mind was dependent on her waistline until she took off the excess weight. Now, she had wonderful nights and wonderful days. Her life was transformed. God had been so good to her. She felt she'd been given a new life. This time, she was determined to take care of it.

Today's thought: Losing weight promises a new lease on life!

September 15

The Lord knoweth how to deliver the godly out of temptations, and to reserve the unjust unto the day of judgment to be punished (2 Peter 2:9).

Woody had a weird dream. His hands and arms got so flabby that he couldn't reach out and pick anything up anymore. Before him stood along table filled with marvelous things to eat, but he was unable to take anything. He woke up sweat-soaked and shuddering. It had seemed so real! He caught a glimpse of himself in the dresser mirror as he sat alone in the night. He was getting awfully plump. Maybe somebody was trying to tell him something. He was no fool. They say that God moves in mysterious ways, and maybe that was true. No reason to push the old luck. Tomorrow the diet begins!

Today's thought: I remember when my eyes could be bigger than my stomach!

September 16

I can do all things through Christ which strengtheneth me (Philippians 4:13).

Jerome stepped up in front of the huge audience. Not too long ago, Jerome wouldn't have been caught dead speaking publicly. All that changed when he found he had something to talk about. Jesus Christ had changed his life, and he wanted the whole world to know. Jerome truly believed that anything was possible for him, now that Jesus Christ was the center of his life.

That same confidence can be ours when we turn our lives over to Jesus. Christ transforms us and enables us to do things that we doubted were possible before. Trust the Lord to help you lose weight, and watch the miracle begin.

Today's thought: I become more spiritually as I become less physically!

September 17

And he said unto me, My grace is sufficient for thee: for my strength is made perfect in weakness. Most gladly therefore will I rather glory in my infirmities, that the power of Christ may rest upon me (2 Corinthians 12:9).

There are times when the hunger pangs get to be almost unbearable. A person gets shaky, she feels weak-kneed and light-headed; it almost feels like an illness. Hunger makes us aware of how really weak we are. A person who is hungry is a person who is humble.

It is good for us to realize that we need help, that we are not always able to stand on our own two feet. In those times of weakness, we learn to rely on the true strength: the power of Jesus Christ. Christ comes to us in our moments of weakness, to strengthen and support us. Praise God that He never lets us fail for very long.

Today's thought: Hunger makes me weak; losing weight makes me strong!

September 18

Let us hold fast the profession of our faith without wavering; (for he is faithful that promised) (Hebrews 10:23).

Kelly believed God would help her. At least, she wanted to believe that God would help. Sometimes she wasn't so sure. She'd begin to doubt, then fear would set in, and she'd comfort herself with a bowl of ice cream or a chocolate bar. Then she'd get mad at herself, she'd pray for help once more, and the whole cycle would start again. If only she could stay convinced that God was with her to give her strength. Kelly knew it wasn't God's fault that she kept giving in. It was her own wavering. Perhaps Kelly's prayer should have been for strength of faith, rather than strength of diet willpower.

Today's thought: I don't think God will help me lose weight; I know it!

September 19
For then shalt thou lift up thy face without spot; yea, thou shalt be stedfast, and shalt not fear (Job 11:15).

What a marvelous feeling, being able to stand up in front of the diet group and tell them she had lost forty-four pounds! Marcie never thought she'd see the day. She remembered all the times when, with great embarrassment, she had to confess that she was not even close to her goal. Those days were behind her. All the doubts and guilt were over. The group had been a great help, too, as God had been. Her faith was a large reason that she was able to stay with it as well as she did. Praise God, everything worked out. She held her head high and shared her great news with the group that had helped her so much.

Today's thought: Doubting never helps get things done!

September 20
He that overcometh shall inherit all things; and I will be his God, and he shall be my son (Revelation 21:7).

Chris thought he was going to die. Why did the gym teacher make the fat kids run track? It wasn't human. His pulse was pounding so hard he thought his eyes might pop out. The finish line looked a million miles away. It wasn't worth it. Somehow he had to lose some of his excess baggage. Nobody could go through life feeling as bad as he presently felt.

We need to overcome our weight problems. Life is not meant to be a struggle, but a blessed gift from God. If we will work to be overcomers, then God will bless our efforts and carry us over the finish line.

Today's thought: With each pound I drop, I move faster toward my goal!

September 21
Surely he shall deliver thee from the snare of the fowler, and from the noisome pestilence (Psalms 91:3).

114

Bert woke up in a cold sweat. He had dreamed that he was lying on a beach, when suddenly the sand began to shift, and he felt himself being sucked downward. Try as he might, he couldn't twist or turn out of the trap. Every way he moved, the sand gave way. He realized that the only reason he was sinking was due to his weight. The more he fought, the deeper he sank. As the sand closed in over his head, he woke up. Quietly, he prayed that the Lord might rescue him from his prison of flesh. Immediately, he was filled with a spirit of sacrifice and commitment equal to the diet that lay before him.

Today's thought: Without a doubt, I'll win this bout!

September 22
Therefore I say unto you, What things soever ye desire, when ye pray, believe that ye receive them, and ye shall have them (Mark 11:24).

Abby knew that God hadn't lost her weight for her, but He sure helped her be able to lose it. When she felt most like giving up, He encouraged her and gave her the will to go on. When she was most tempted to break her diet, He reminded her of how important it was to stick with it. When the pounds began to fall, He filled her with a deep joy that insured she would continue. She never forgot to pray, whether it was for help, for strength, or for thanksgiving. Abby hadn't lost the weight all by herself. God helped more than she could ever know.

Today's thought: I'm glad that I'm a loser . . . of weight!

September 23
God is our refuge and strength, a very present help in trouble (Psalms 46:1).

Barb hated it when her husband went away on business trips. He was her conscience when it came to watching what she ate. Besides, when she was lonely she had the tendency to eat to compensate. It was so much harder to diet when he went away.

It is good to know that we have a refuge and strength that never goes on vacation. God is ever with us, and He will help us whenever we need Him. When the temptations are the greatest, then we can be confident that God will be the strongest.

Today's thought: I will turn to God when my diet gets too tough!

September 24
But let him ask in faith, nothing wavering. For he that wavereth is like a wave of the sea driven with the wind and tossed (James 1:6).

Sybil couldn't understand why Bev kept praying about her diet. It seemed so silly. Sybil was a good Christian, but she didn't bother talking about such trivial things with God. God had much better things to do than watch people lose weight, didn't He? Still, Bev seemed to be doing much better on her diet than Sybil was. Bev didn't struggle with temptation as much, and she was much better at saying no when she was offered rich, fattening foods. Maybe Bev had something. Her prayers were obviously a help to her, and Sybil had nothing to lose but her weight. Sybil decided to ask Bev for some guidance.

Today's thought: Too much doubt rules weight loss out!

September 25
The name of the Lord is a strong tower: the righteous runneth into it, and is safe (Proverbs 18:10).

Every few weeks or so, Ellen would go off by herself to her grandmother's farm for a day alone. She would fast for the entire day, and each time hunger would overtake her, she would pause to pray to God. She thanked Him for providing her with food and sustenance through the week. She thanked Him for her life in a country where she was free to do what she wanted to. She thanked Him that she didn't have to struggle day to day for survival. The times on the farm meant so much to her. Ellen found great strength in those times when hunger made her feel so weak. It was good to take time to be thankful.

Today's thought: I'll try not to think of what I don't have, but what I do have!

September 26
Fear not: for I am with thee: I will bring thy seed from the east, and gather thee from the west (Isaiah 43:5).

It didn't look like it was going to work out. Becky wanted to lose a few pounds before the dance. It wasn't any big deal, but that made it worse. She'd had almost six weeks, and in that time she hadn't lost any weight at all. She kept telling herself she had plenty of time, but time had slipped away. Now it was too late, and she felt terrible. Why had she been so stupid? Why hadn't she taken it more seriously? Not only did she feel bad because she was overweight, but she also felt guilty and hopeless. Somehow she had to learn to knuckle down and stick to what she needed to do. With God's help, maybe she could.

Today's thought: Today I lose weight; tomorrow's too late!

September 27

And they that know thy name will put their trust in thee: for thou, Lord, hast not forsaken them that seek thee (Psalms 9:10).

It was nice to see that the church cared so much about the ladies' group that dieted together. At the annual church planning board dinner, it was suggested that a low-calorie menu be offered. Dieting was so much easier when other people understood and cooperated with you. It was gratifying to be supported by the church as if by one's own family. God had been good to the ladies of the church.

God's love should be apparent in our churches. The church should be a place where we know we will be affirmed and supported. God never forsakes His children, and His children should be careful not to forsake each other.

Today's thought: No matter what, I'm not in this diet alone!

September 28

For I the Lord thy God will hold thy right hand, saying unto thee, Fear not; I will help thee (Isaiah 41:13).

When Jenny was young, her mother used to hold her hand whenever she was afraid or worried. Just the feel of her mother's hand in hers gave her strength and courage. There were days when Jenny wished her mom was close enough to hold hands with, but she lived hundreds of miles away. She especially wanted her mother's support now that she was dieting. Whenever things got particularly tough, she would close her eyes to say a short prayer. As she prayed, she imagined her hand in Jesus' hand, and she felt a wonderful peace and comfort. That image gave Jenny all the strength she needed.

Today's thought: I'm never too heavy for God to pick up!

September 29

These things I have spoken unto you, that in me ye might have peace. In the world ye shall have tribulation: but be of good cheer; I have overcome the world (John 16:33).

Leo wanted to remember how tough it was. He'd lost the weight, but he never wanted to get back into the poor shape he'd recently been in. It would be way too easy to fall back into bad habits, thinking that the battle was won once for all time. It was nice to have succeeded. But Leo planned to make sure his success lasted a good, long time.

It is nice to overcome obesity, but it is an ongoing battle. We should ally ourselves with the one true conqueror: Jesus Christ. With Christ's help, we can continue to triumph over our weight problems. He grants not only peace, but power to overcome any obstacle.

Today's thought: If we empty our plate, we won't lose our weight!

September 30

Wait on the Lord: be of good courage, and he shall strengthen thine heart: wait, I say, on the Lord (Psalms 27:14).

Kerri wished she could lose weight just a little bit faster. She really didn't have anything to complain about. Since she started her diet, she had consistently lost. There were days, though, when she simply got tired of dieting. She doubted whether she was ever going to lose the weight she wanted to lose. All those times, she turned to God for encouragement. Talking to the Lord always made Kerri feel better. She really believed that He knew what she was going through. If God could be patient with her when she complained about her diet, she figured she could be more patient as she attempted to lose weight.

Today's thought: Without patience, I'll never lose weight!

OCTOBER
Strength

When we diet, we learn quickly how truly weak we are. It takes great strength to diet: strength of will, strength of character, strength of mind. It takes a great deal of wisdom to admit that we don't possess all the strength we need on our own. Somehow we need to tap into a greater source of strength. That source is Jesus Christ the Lord. His strength never wavers, never fails. He has strength great enough to conquer death itself. The amazing thing about the strength of Christ is that it is freely offered to everyone who asks for it. When we feel the weakest, that is when we are most open to the strength of Christ. Call upon the Lord, and He will be quick to answer. Reach out for His strength, and you will find yourself able to conquer your weight problem better than you could ever hope to on your own. Our God is a God of strength and power. Hallelujah!

October 1
Therefore I take pleasure in infirmities, in reproaches, in necessities, in persecutions, in distresses for Christ's sake: for when I am weak, then am I strong (2 Corinthians 12:10).

Having to diet was like having a bad rash. It was almost impossible to ignore, and it never went away. It was a real test of will not to give in when the stomach started growling. More than anything else, it was infuriating to feel so weak. It wasn't that he was starving. He ate regularly, just not as much as he was used to. He always prided himself on being a strong person. His diet was proving otherwise. He was short-tempered and cranky. As hard as it was, he had to admit he needed help. He prayed for God to strengthen him through his diet. With God's help, he felt he might just make it.

Today's thought: I'm stronger than my stomach gives me credit for being!

October 2
Wherefore take unto you the whole armour of God, that ye may be able to withstand in the evil day, and having done all, to stand (Ephesians 6:13).

Even the mightiest warrior of old was not foolish enough to enter battle without protection. Strength must be tempered with common sense. When we wage war on fat, we need to be well equipped for the fray. If we give something up, we need to have something to replace it with. Jesus proposed that we should not live by bread only, but upon the word of God. We can protect ourselves from temptation by faith. God will fight our battle alongside us. With Christ, we become an invincible army. We can carry on in the strength of the Spirit, which will allow us to conquer our weight and fears. With Christ comes true power.

Today's thought: With Jesus' might, my fat I'll fight!

October 3

The righteous also shall hold on his way, and he that hath clean hands should be stronger and stronger (Job 17:9).

Mort juggled his folder of papers, his coffee, and his sweet roll. It seemed as though Mort couldn't go anywhere without his hands full of food. Even now, as he rushed toward an important meeting, he fed his face. As he rounded the corner, a great gust of wind took him by surprise, ripping the folder from his hands. The sheets of his report flew off in many directions as he watched helplessly, sweet roll in hand. Looking at the messy roll clutched in his fingers, he silently swore to cut out all the snacks. Not only were they ruining his body, but now they jeopardized his job. It just wasn't worth it.

Today's thought: I don't want my greatest skill to be my ability to eat!

October 4

Not that I speak in respect of want: for I have learned, in whatsoever state I am, therewith to be content (Philippians 4:11).

Sam remembered the P.O.W. camp he had spent six years in. Whenever he began to feel sorry for himself as he dieted, he remembered the time in his life when he really had something to be upset about. Dieting was nothing, compared to the hell he had suffered through. It humbled him a little. He gained great strength from the memory. God had gotten him through the war, so he knew God could get him through the diet. As long as he had the memory of all he had come through before, he knew he could make it through anything else that came his way.

Today's thought: God brings me through every situation, whether large or small.

October 5

I will lift up mine eyes unto the hills, from whence cometh my help. My help cometh from the Lord, which made heaven and earth (Psalms 121:1, 2).

Sonya was just about to dip into the ice cream when her doorbell rang. Guiltily, she threw the container into the freezer and slammed the door. Rushing to the hallway, she opened the door and found her sister standing there. Time after time, her sister showed up when she was most needed. Sonya couldn't believe the number of times her sister had been there to help her resist temptation. Sonya felt God was really watching out for her. Whenever her own strength gave out, God sent someone along who could strengthen her. Relieved, she let her sister in and told her the service she had just performed.

Today's thought: Strength comes from unexpected places when our own gives out!

October 6

But they that wait upon the Lord shall renew their strength; they shall mount up with wings as eagles; they shall run, and not be weary; and they shall walk, and not faint (Isaiah 40:31).

Kip was amazed at how easily he took the stairs. When his kids had begged him to climb to the top of the Statue of Liberty with them, he had squirmed. He remembered what a labor it had been when he was fat. He knew that he never would have made it before. Instead of a painful trauma, he found the climb a relative breeze. Thank God he had been able to lose the weight. It was the best move he ever made. It had been tough, but Kip had relied heavily on God to help him out. While he had been dieting, he had needed God's strength. Now that he was thin, God let him use his own strength once again.

Today's thought: Food gives us temporary strength. God gives us strength forever!

October 7

But we are not of them who draw back unto perdition; but of them that believe to the saving of the soul (Hebrews 10:39).

Darren felt bad withdrawing from the group, but he had to. The other three men kept cheating on their diets, and that was no help at all. Each time they gave in to temptation, Darren asked himself why he tried so hard when everyone else quit. Darren needed strength and support, not more temptation. At least on his own he stood a fighting chance. Darren prayed for guidance. Dieting was hard enough without other people making it harder.

We need to attach ourselves to those who are serious and committed to losing weight. God will help us have all the strength we need to keep on our diets.

Today's thought: The weight that I've lost, was of minimal cost!

October 8
Behold also the ships, which though they be so great, and are driven of fierce winds, yet are they turned about with a very small helm, whithersoever the governor listeth (James 3:4).

David Gregory spoke to groups all over the country. He believed that faith could help people achieve all their goals. He spoke to weight-loss groups in particular, because he had once been grossly overweight, and it had been his faith that had brought him through. Often, people would skeptically confront him as to how he really lost all his weight. His answer never varied. When asked, he would produce a tiny pewter cross from his pocket. All his success, all his power, all his wealth were nothing, compared to the strength of that small symbol. The power of the cross of Christ is unequalled.

Today's thought: With each little loss of weight, I make a greater gain!

October 9
Trust ye in the Lord for ever: for in the Lord JEHOVAH is everlasting strength (Isaiah 26:4).

Lettuce! Celery! Lowfat cottage cheese! Yeesh! It never got any more interesting. The same old bland foods got tiresome after awhile. Debbie thought she would go crazy before long. She knew what she was doing was a good thing. She really wanted to lose weight. She wanted to look and feel great. Sometimes she didn't know whether it was going to pay off. She believed that God was happy with her desire to lose weight. She trusted that He would help her. Often, it was only the strength she received from trying to please God that kept her going. She was thankful that God gave her that kind of strength.

Today's thought: The only thing I'll give up is being fat!

October 10
Is any among you afflicted? let him pray. Is any merry? let him sing psalms (James 5:13).

Bill kept telling June to ask God for help. June couldn't quite bring herself to do it. Prayer was for weaklings. Only people who couldn't handle life prayed. June would rather struggle by on her own than rely on a crutch.

False pride is a sad affliction. People who feel that they are strong enough to handle every situation of life only fool themselves. Everyone is weak at some point in her life. The truly strong person is the one who acknowledges her weakness and has the wisdom to turn to God for help.

Today's thought: More time in prayer means less time to eat!

October 11
And who is he that will harm you, if ye be followers of that which is good? (1 Peter 3:13.)

Kim's mother felt so sorry for her. She remembered what it was like to be overweight. All the other children were so cruel. She could still feel the sting of all the nicknames people put on her. Now, Kim was suffering the same indignities. Her mother hoped she could get Kim on a diet, if for no other reason than to keep Kim's classmates from taunting her so mercilessly. Just taking steps to correct the problem made it easier to take. The insults didn't hurt so much after the problem was taken care of. Together, they would lose the weight. With God's help, time would heal the wounds of unkind words.

Today's thought: I will put all my excess weight behind me!

October 12
But as many as received him, to them gave he power to become the sons of God, even to them that believe on his name (John 1:12).

Corey had to admit that his friends were making better progress than he was. He just wasn't disciplined enough. His friends didn't seem to have nearly as much trouble with discipline. When he asked them why, they all just grinned and told him to pray about it. Finally, it dawned on him what they were talking about. Corey wasn't much of a Christian, but he wasn't stupid, either. His friends obviously had something he needed and wanted. If God could do so much to help them, then Corey believed He would do it for him, also. By receiving the truth of Christ, Corey was given all the strength needed to succeed in his diet.

Today's thought: God is ready to help me lose weight!

October 13
Submit yourselves therefore to God. Resist the devil, and he will flee from you (James 4:7).

Grace was surprised. The hostess had offered her dessert and she had declined without even the slightest pang of remorse. Dessert had always been Grace's favorite. Giving up dessert had been the worst part of her diet. Now, though, she found that she had declined without really caring. What a breakthrough! She felt she had a fighting chance. She had resisted temptation so long that it wasn't tempting any longer. Grace felt stronger than at any other point in her diet. Thank God. She was going to make it, after all!

Today's thought: The more I turn down, the more my weight goes down!

October 14

Wherefore let him that thinketh he standeth take heed lest he fall (1 Corinthians 10:12).

Peter dressed for the dinner. His friends tried to tell him he shouldn't go, but he ignored them. He'd been doing great on his diet. He was in total control. He knew there would be wonderful and exotic food where he was going, but he could handle it. Too bad he forgot that when he got there. The temptation was too great for him. Before he realized what was happening, he was stuffed. In one day, he blew a couple of weeks of hard work.

We can't afford to get cocky when we diet. Each day is a new struggle all its own. Ask God for daily help. Avoid situations where temptation prevails. The Lord will be sure to help you, whenever you let Him.

Today's thought: I will steer clear of calorie traps!

October 15

Then he answered and spake unto me, saying, This is the word of the Lord unto Zerubbabel, saying, Not by might, nor by power, but by my spirit, saith the Lord of hosts (Zechariah 4:6).

Curtis liked to think he could do everything on his own. He often told friends that he didn't need anybody else; he was fine all by himself. On those rare occasions when Curt was feeling down and in need of a friend's support, he usually found himself alone. Everyone figured he really didn't need anyone else, and so he was lonely.

No matter how strong or powerful or talented we might be, we all need the support of friends. Our greatest friend is, of course, Jesus Christ. We need never feel alone when we have the Spirit of the Lord with us. Accept the helping hand of the Lord, and find out what real strength is all about.

Today's thought: Let me lose not only weight, but also false pride!

October 16

Jesus answered, Thou couldest have no power at all against me, except it were given thee from above: therefore he that delivered me unto thee hath the greater sin (John 19:11).

How much easier our lives would be if we could quit fighting the fact that all power comes from God. We want control of our own lives, and we like to think we can stand on our own two feet. The reality of the matter is that we have received everything we have from the Lord. He has given us our abilities and talents, He has given us our resources, and He gives us our opportunities. The truly strong person is she who understands that God is the source of all power. If we want the power to diet, it can come to us only through the Lord God Almighty, who loves His children and offers them everything they need.

Today's thought: God is greater than my desire to eat!

October 17

But speaking the truth in love, may grow up into him in all things, which is the head, even Christ: from whom the whole body fitly joined together and compacted by that which every joint supplieth, according to the effectual working in the measure of every part, maketh increase of the body unto the edifying of itself in love (Ephesians 4:15, 16).

Peak efficiency: That is what God intended for the human body. The human body is an intricate, delicate, but powerful machine; finely crafted, and capable of amazing feats. The only way the body can work properly, the way God intended, is when we take good care of it. It should not be burdened with excessive weight, nor should it be abused by improper diet. If we will endeavor to take good care of our bodies, we will experience the joy of living the way God intended for us all.

Today's thought: I am a marvelous creation of God, worth taking care of!

October 18

O God, thou art terrible out of thy holy places: the God of Israel is he that giveth strength and power unto his people. Blessed be God (Psalms 68:35).

Theo knew the power of God. He had seen it in the birth of his daughter. He had felt it when his father had died. He had witnessed it many times in the glorious creation of nature. Theo had no doubt about the power of God. He had worked in forestry for his entire life. He had flown through thunderstorms where lightning splintered huge trees and set forests blazing. The power of God was both a wondeful and a terrifying thing. Theo had no doubt that there was nothing beyond the power of God. The God of all creation could handle his diet. He had no question in his mind. Strength such as God's was a good thing to have on his side!

Today's thought: With God on my side, my fat doesn't stand a chance!

October 19

Moreover when ye fast, be not, as the hypocrites, of a sad countenance: for they disfigure their faces, that they may appear unto men to fast. Verily I say unto you, They have their reward (Matthew 6:16).

Everyone knew enough to stay out of Kevin's way when he was on a diet. The man became a raving lunatic. He couldn't get along with anybody. Connie felt he acted that way just to let everyone know he was on a diet. Then, when he gave up on it, nobody had the nerve to suggest he give it another try. It was his way of justifying not having to diet. Connie just wished he'd quit putting on such performances. it made everyone else miserable.

Our diets need to be our business, unless we turn to others for help. We diet for the wrong reasons if all we want is sympathy or attention. God will give strength to those who are sincere, but He is unable to help those who really don't want help.

Today's thought: My diet will not become a burden to anyone else!

October 20

But the God of all grace, who hath called us unto his eternal glory by Christ Jesus, after that ye have suffered a while, make you perfect, stablish, strengthen, settle you (1 Peter 5:10).

Cliff felt content. He felt good about the diet. He knew it was time to do something, so it didn't feel like such a great struggle. He prayed for God's help, and he felt God's presence with him. Sure, there would be unpleasantness, as there was whenever a sacrifice was involved, but it would all be well worth it. The prospect of being healthy and trim was very appealing to him. Cliff had confidence that God would bless him with strength, courage, and peace. With that kind of assurance, how could he go wrong?

Today's thought: If God will give me everything I really need, how can I help but lose weight?

October 21

Another parable put he forth unto them, saying, The kingdom of heaven is like to a grain of mustard seed, which a man took, and sowed in his field: which indeed is the least of all seeds: but when it is grown, it is the greatest among herbs, and becometh a tree, so that the birds of the air come and lodge in the branches thereof (Matthew 13:31, 32).

All too often, people tackle diets that are too big for them. They try to give up everything at once, hoping to lose a huge amount of weight in a short period of time. Usually, that won't work. We should learn that the greatest successes come in small steps. We need to set modest goals that we can handle, so we don't get discouraged. God blesses our small efforts, for they are usually the most sincere and realistic. Ask God's guidance, and He will grant you exactly the right amount of strength you need to triumph.

Today's thought: Giving up a little at a time will keep me from giving up altogether!

October 22

Who is weak, and I am not weak? who is offended, and I burn not? If I must needs glory, I will glory of the things which concern mine infirmities (2 Corinthians 11:29, 30).

If there was one thing to respect Cynthia for, it was her humility. She was very talented, but she knew well what she could do and what she couldn't. She was never shy about asking for help when she needed it, and she never tried to make people think she could do things she could not. It was nice to see someone who could admit her weaknesses without being defensive or insecure. When Cynthia had dieted, she openly admitted that she relied heavily on God for strength and encouragement. It was a real inspiration to others to find someone who gained strength from being honest about weakness.

Today's thought: It is more important to be strong of heart than strong of body!

October 23

Thou hast thrust sore at me that I might fall: but the Lord helped me. The Lord is my strength and song, and is become my salvation (Psalms 118:13, 14).

Going home to Mother's was murder on the diet. Stacy dreaded it. She knew the minute she walked in, her mother would ask her why she wasn't eating right, and then, for the next week, her mother would shove fattening, although delicious, dishes in front of her face. Going home required a double measure of strength. At those times, Stacy had to pray doubly hard. Sometimes it worked, sometimes she gave in. In the end, though, Stacy was glad to have God to turn to. Once back in her own apartment, He gave her all the resolve she needed to get right back on her diet. Truly, the Lord was her strength and her salvation.

Today's thought: I need saving from that which I would devour!

October 24

Fear thou not; for I am with thee: be not dismayed; for I am thy God: I will strengthen thee; yea, I will help thee; yea, I will uphold thee with the right hand of my righteousness (Isaiah 41:10).

The evening was the worst. About an hour before bedtime, Eleanor would begin to get cravings. The worst possible thing to do would be to eat right before bed. Sometimes her stomach would growl so much that she thought she would wake up the neighborhood. On those occasions, Eleanor asked God for a little quick relief and went straight to bed. Better that than to pig out and feel lousy the rest of the night and guilty all the following day! God can grant us blessed relief from the whinings of the stomach. He can take our mind off our stomachs and give us the strength to say no!

Today's thought: The waistline won't grow if I learn to say no!

October 25

Take my yoke upon you, and learn of me; for I am meek and lowly in heart: and ye shall find rest unto your souls. For my yoke is easy, and my burden is light (Matthew 11:29, 30).

The most impressive thing about Laura was that no one realized she was on her diet. She never complained. She never made a big deal about what she could and couldn't eat. She never whined around or moped, hoping someone would ask her what was the matter. She just quietly, patiently lost weight. The rest of the women in the office were astonished. Laura made it seem so easy. Laura just smiled at all their comments, content to know that God had helped her be strong when she needed Him. There had been many times when Laura would have liked to complain or mope, but each time God had rallied her spirits and helped her get by.

Today's thought: During my diet, I'll smile even when I feel like crying!

October 26

Forasmuch then as Christ hath suffered for us in the flesh, arm yourselves likewise with the same mind: for he that hath suffered in the flesh hath ceased from sin; that he no longer should live the rest of his time in the flesh to the lusts of men, but to the will of God (1 Peter 4:1, 2).

128

Barney knew he could lose weight. He'd given up cigarettes, and that was the hardest thing he'd ever had to do. If he could do away with cigarettes, he was positive he could lose weight. A friend had once told him that if he was suffering, he knew he was on the right track. Nothing worth doing came easy. Barney asked God for strength as he set about losing weight. When he felt he was suffering the most, that's when he relied most heavily on God. A little suffering never hurt anyone, especially when it was done in order to attain good health.

Today's thought: I suffer now so that I can enjoy the rest of my life!

October 27
Wherefore lift up the hands which hang down, and the feeble knees (Hebrews 12:12).

Monica hated evenings that she had to spend alone. When she was with friends, she felt so much stronger. She put forth all her energy to have a good time when she went out. On the nights she stayed home, however, she just didn't have the strength to put on a happy front. Dieting was so much more difficult without help from friends.

It is good to know that God is ever with us. On those occasions when there is no one around to help us, we can turn to God for strength and endurance. He helps us pick ourselves up and continue on our way. He strengthens feeble knees and lifts hands that hang down.

Today's thought: My energy comes from a source other than food!

October 28
Confess your faults one to another, and pray one for another, that ye may be healed. The effectual fervent prayer of a righteous man availeth much (James 5:16).

The best idea the group ever had was to pray for one another. Every Monday morning, they got together for exercise and a Bible study. They talked about their diets and how things were going, and they had to announce publicly what their weight was and how much they had lost or gained. Then, they promised to pray for one another, and they swapped telephone numbers so they could give a call of encouragement through the week. It was a wonderful system, and it helped so much to know you weren't dieting alone. The power of a well-meant prayer was amazing. It made dieting much easier.

Today's thought: A prayer a day keeps the flabbies away!

October 29

Then he said unto them, Go your way, eat the fat, and drink the sweet, and send portions unto them for whom nothing is prepared: for this day is holy unto our Lord: neither be ye sorry: for the joy of the Lord is your strength (Nehemiah 8:10).

Patrick always hated programs on starving people around the world. The minute they would come on, he would turn off the television. What business was it of his if people halfway around the world were starving? He had all he needed, and he worked hard for it. So what if he was overweight? He earned that right because he was born in America!

The Bible teaches us that God gives us an abundance for just one reason: So that we will share it with those in need. If we take the bounty God offers and are selfish or gluttonous with it, then we are saying to God that we won't live as His children. We should take only what we need, and share the rest, for that is the way of God.

Today's thought: I have more than I need, and I don't really need much of what I want.

October 30

But the salvation of the righteous is of the Lord: he is their strength in the time of trouble (Psalms 37:39).

Bob had a terrible dream. Food kept coming at him from every direction. Wherever it touched him, it stuck to him. Before long he couldn't move. He had trouble breathing. He had trouble seeing. He was hot and slimy. He kept trying to reach out for help, but no help came. He was buried under a mountain of food. As he lay awake thinking of the dream, he realized that it wasn't far from the truth. He was buried by a mountain of food become flesh. He did have trouble breathing and moving. It wasn't worth it. Silently, he reached out for help in a meek and humble prayer. God, the source of salvation, reached back.

Today's thought: God, save me from an appetite seldom satisfied!

October 31

Do all things without murmurings and disputings: that ye may be blameless and harmless, the sons of God, without rebuke, in the midst of a crooked and perverse nation, among whom ye shine as lights in the world (Philippians 2:14, 15).

Peggy kept looking at her daughter's trick-or-treat bag. Her daughter had made a grand haul of chocolates and sugary candies. It was all Peg could do to keep her hands off it. A little devil inside kept telling her that her daughter wouldn't miss a few pieces. Peggy wanted to dive in so badly it hurt. She walked over to the bag and looked in. On its own, her hand moved toward the sweets. She was about to grab a handful when a still small voice stopped her. What had she been trying to teach her daughter about honesty and respecting things that weren't hers? Now she was attempting to pilfer her daughter's trick-or-treat bag because she wanted candy. When would she ever learn some strength and self-restraint?

Today's thought: I will avoid things that make me less of a person, but more of a body!

NOVEMBER
Joy and Thanksgiving

Those who are in captivity learn to truly understand the value of freedom. When we have been captive to an abundance of flesh, we long for freedom from obesity. To be able to walk any distance without feeling exhausted, to be able to wear fashionable clothing, to look fit, to not be embarrassed; all these things attain a precious value when we don't have them. When we travel the road toward a healthy, normal body, we come to appreciate the gift of the human form that God intended us to have. We learn to be thankful for what we have been given, and when we live as God intended us to live, we come to possess a deep and abiding joy beyond words. God gave us life to enjoy to the fullest. When we allow our bodies to become unfit, we make it impossible to live life as fully as is possible. Our Lord offers us a second chance; a chance to renew ourselves and enter into a life of peace and joy. Let us be thankful that He loves us enough to help us find a truly fulfilling life.

November 1

For God is not unrighteous to forget your work and labour of love, which ye have shewed toward his name, in that ye have ministered to the saints, and do minister (Hebrews 6:10).

What a great reward! Robin had never looked so good. All her months of dieting paid off royally. It was beautiful to see the expressions on people's faces when they saw her. She couldn't wait to go out to show herself off. God had certainly blessed her through the rough time of dieting. There were days when she decided it just wasn't worth it. Now, she could hardly believe she ever had doubts. Looking in the mirror, she even surprised herself. She never thought she'd look this good.

When we dedicate ourselves to doing things that are right and good to do, God is sure to bless us and reward us for our labors.

Today's thought: Improvement comes with practice. I can even get good at dieting!

133

November 2

My brethren, count it all joy when ye fall into divers temptations (James 1:2).

Renee really felt good whenever she had the strength to say no to food that was offered to her. Each time she could refuse eating, it made her feel she'd won a moral victory. Mentally, she kept score. It became a game to see how often she could hold out between defeats. In a strange way, it made her diet enjoyable. She felt she was really accomplishing something that was important. By the end of about four months, Renee was able to defeat just about every temptation that came along. She felt God's pleasure as she grew more able to decline treats. That joy made her diet fly by.

Today's thought: Diets can be fun, especially when they're done!

November 3

He that goeth forth and weepeth, bearing precious seed, shall doubtless come again with rejoicing, bringing his sheaves with him (Psalms 126:6).

The groaning was over. The long nights of hunger lay behind. For some strange reason, the diet was getting easier. Finally, Diane's body had gotten the message that snacks and heavy meals were no more. The cravings and cryings of her stomach subsided. It had been a tough war, but Diane felt she had scored a victory at long last. All the weeping was behind, and she felt a wonderful joy. She knew that plenty of tough times lay ahead, but she also knew she could handle them. With God's help, she would make it. The hardest part was behind her.

Today's thought: When I take it one day at a time, the days fall away as fast as the pounds!

November 4

Likewise, I say unto you, there is joy in the presence of the angels of God over one sinner that repenteth (Luke 15:10).

Paul fumbled with his keys outside his apartment. When he tried the lock, the door swung inward. Cautiously, he entered. As he switched on the light, a dozen of his friends and neighbors jumped out, shouting, "Surprise!" They had come out to offer a congratulations party for the sixty pounds Paul had been able to lose. It was such a wonderful moment. Paul had felt joyful about what he had done for some time, but it was something special to have friends celebrate with him. God had blessed Paul so much. Not only had He helped him when he dieted, but He gave him such good friends.

Today's thought: To gain means starvation; to lose, jubilation!

November 5

Blessed are ye, when men shall revile you, and persecute you, and shall say all manner of evil against you falsely, for my sake (Matthew 5:11).

Ken could hardly wait to get back to school. Peter had ridden him about his weight the entire year before. When Ken had vowed to lose weight over the summer, Pete had laughed at him. "Fat boy, you can't keep away from the food. You'll be back, big as a beach ball. Don't kid yourself!"

Ken could hardly wait to make Pete eat those words. He had spent the entire summer as a Christian youth counselor at camp. The people there were so supportive of what he was trying to do. They had made it possible. Not only had they helped him lose weight, but they helped him show Peter just how wrong he could be!

Today's thought: I'm going to prove that there's more to me than my weight!

November 6

And Jesus stood still, and commanded him to be called. And they call the blind man, saying unto him, Be of good comfort, rise; he calleth thee. And he, casting away his garment, rose, and came to Jesus (Mark 10:49, 50).

Kate was so thankful. God had truly blessed her. She had been on the verge of collapse, and the doctor told her that her weight had to go. Reluctantly, she had started to diet, not expecting any great results. She prayed for God to help her, because she felt so weak. When the doctor gave her a clean bill of health, she closed her eyes and prayed.

God is God of the impossible. When we say "can't," He says "can." Faith is believing that God can, and will, help us when we are in need. God cares for His children, and for that we should be eternally grateful.

Today's thought: I'd rather be grateful than have another plateful!

November 7

But my God shall supply all your need according to his riches in glory by Christ Jesus (Philippians 4:19).

It really wasn't fair that so many thin people couldn't understand what it meant to be fat. Patty got mad when skinny friends chastised her for not sticking to her diet better. What did they know? Patty was always so thankful to God for what weight she'd been able to lose already that she could never understand why her friends put her down. Didn't they know what she had to sacrifice?

Whenever Patty got mad at her friends, she asked Got to help calm her down. His peace filled her heart, and she was able to relax. God had done so much for her while she dieted. Too bad her friends couldn't see it.

Today's thought: God is with me when it feels like the world is against me!

November 8

For what thanks can we render to God again for you, for all the joy wherewith we joy for your sakes before our God (1 Thessalonians 3:9).

Gail wished she could do more for Mrs. Cooper. One night Mrs. Cooper had passed by her apartment and heard Gail crying. She stopped to see if there was anything she could do to help. Gail told her about her diet and how hard it was. Mrs. Cooper had been very sympathetic, and had spent many hours with her since. She helped take Gail's mind off food. Gail really felt strongly that she wouldn't have made it through the diet without Mrs. Cooper.

We have someone who will listen to us when things get to be too much for us. That someone is God, and we can be thankful that He is ever with us, ready to listen to the concerns of our hearts.

Today's thought: Let your praises to God be louder than the grumblings of your stomach!

November 9

. . . Naked came I out of my mother's womb, and naked shall I return thither: the Lord gave, and the Lord hath taken away; blessed be the name of the Lord (Job 1:21).

Stella was extremely frustrated. She had worked so hard to lose weight. She had done a great job, but now it was even harder to keep it off. She felt she was doing a good job of eating the right foods in small quantities, but when she'd step on the scales, she would find her weight creeping up. She always thought that once she got her weight down, everything would be easy. Boy, was that false! Weight-watching was a full-time job! Stella used to pray for God to keep her in line, but now the prayers were needed all the time. It just went to prove that nothing could be taken for granted. Good things don't come easy, but they're still worth having.

Today's thought: Lord, give me strength, but take my weight problem!

November 10

And he answered and said unto them, I tell you that, if these should hold their peace, the stones would immediately cry out (Luke 19:40).

Preston could hardly contain his excitement as the plane approached its landing. He hadn't seen his sister in over a year. At their last meeting he had weighed about 260 pounds. Now, he was a trim 180. He couldn't wait to see her face. He never remembered being so anxious to see anyone before in his life. It was important to him to please his family, and he knew nothing would please his sister more than to see him looking so good.

God gives us such experiences to make our sacrifices worthwhile. We can be thankful that God motivates us in such loving ways. With His blessed help, we can't keep from succeeding.

Today's thought: I want others to see me like they've never seen me before!

November 11

Again, the kingdom of heaven is like unto treasure hid in a field; the which when a man hath found, he hideth, and for joy thereof goeth and selleth all that he hath, and buyeth that field (Matthew 13:44).

Kris would give anything to be thin again. She was willing to diet, she was willing to exercise, she was willing to try anything. Following a number of traumatic experiences in her life, she had let herself go, but now she regretted it with all her heart. Earnestly she began to pray to God. Within a few weeks, her dieting was beginning to pay off. Delighted with the results, she doubled her efforts, with her doctor's permission, and devoted herself to her diet, body, mind, and soul. For the first time in years, she found herself happy and content. The joy she found was a blessed gift from God.

Today's thought: I'm looking for little victories to keep me dieting!

November 12

I thank my God, making mention of thee always in my prayers, that the communication of thy faith may become effectual by the acknowledging of every good thing which is in you in Christ Jesus (Philemon 1:4, 6).

Thomas was a great help with members of the group. He had lost so much weight, on more than one occasion, so he knew what it was like to triumph as well as to fall back into failure. He had rallied, though, and beaten his weight problem again. He was living proof that it could be done, and that it wasn't hopeless when temptation got the better of a person. He shared his story with many people, and he helped them through some hard struggles. He was a faithful man, and his faith shone through. God had called Thomas to a very special ministry, and he answered that call in a very special way.

Today's thought: I may fall back time and again, but I'm heading in the right direction!

November 13
Whom having not seen, ye love; in whom, though now ye see him not, yet believing, ye rejoice with joy unspeakable and full of glory: receiving the end of your faith, even the salvation of your souls (1 Peter 1:8, 9).

Stephanie always had a picture of what she would look like in the back of her mind. She used to dream of how she would look once she lost weight. It was hard to imagine, but she did it anyway. That image in her mind kept her going through some rough spots. Her dream gave her motivation. Though she didn't really know what she'd look like, her imagination kept her on the right path.

Faith means acting on what we believe, even when we can't actually see the object of our faith. Faith in God teaches us how to put faith in action. When we are motivated by what we do not yet see, we find strength and joy in the living of our lives.

Today's thought: In my mind I see a whole new me!

November 14
Looking unto Jesus the author and finisher of our faith; who for the joy that was set before him endured the cross, despising the shame, and is set down at the right hand of the throne of God (Hebrews 12:2).

Mary took comfort from the gospels. Whenever she felt sorry for herself, she looked at the Bible. She couldn't believe all that Jesus had done and suffered. He had so much, and He emptied Himself to give to others. In the end, He received eternal glory. What a wonderful lesson. Dieting is a temporary and comparatively minor sacrifice, compared with Christ. And yet, as Christ triumphed over His situation, so shall we triumph over ours. Christ is our example in all things. The author and finisher of our faith has shown us the way to victory, and we share in His joy when we triumph in our own lives.

Today's thought: What I suffer today is worth the victory tomorrow!

November 15
For he that is mighty hath done to me great things; and holy is

his name (Luke 1:49).

Al sat in his chair, looking around the living room at all the people he loved so much. Six months ago, he had almost died of a heart attack. Today he was forty pounds trimmer and a whole lot healthier. He had so much to be thankful for. God had been so good to him. He never realized how much life meant to him until he almost lost it. Now he found it wasn't that hard to watch his diet and his blood pressure. It was worth it. God had done great things for Al. The least he could do was take good care of himself. After all, he had a great family that he planned to enjoy into his old, old age.

Today's thought: Life is a gift from God that I have no right to abuse!

November 16
Praise ye the Lord. Praise the Lord, O my soul. The Lord openeth the eyes of the blind: the Lord raiseth them that are bowed down: the Lord loveth the righteous (Psalms 146:1, 8).

Dick couldn't believe everyone was against him. First, his wife started making comments about his weight. Next, it was his doctor. Now, his friends at the office. Lord, he looked the same as he always did. Why was everyone picking on him all of the sudden? Maybe he had gained a little, but that was just normal spread for a middle-aged man. He'd never worried about weight before, and he sure wasn't planning to start worrying now.

Sometimes we are too blind to see when we need to lose weight. Pride gets in the way, and we aren't honest with ourselves. Ask God to help keep ego out of the way, and He will open your eyes to see what needs to be done.

Today's thought: When it comes to weight, I won't kid myself!

November 17
Sing unto the Lord; for he hath done excellent things: this is known in all the earth (Isaiah 12:5).

Ann went out shopping for a whole new winter wardrobe. Everyday of her diet, she had put money away for just this very day. She had set a goal for herself, and she promised to take herself shopping when she reached it. Now was that day, and she was overjoyed. For the first time in years, she wasn't embarrassed to go out for new things. She could walk into normal stores and pull things off the rack to wear. She could find new fashions and not worry about whether they came in her size. The whole world looked brighter. God had been so good to her, and she was thankful. Now she was going to be good to herself!

Today's thought: I'm going to treat myself to a new me!

November 18

And immediately he received his sight, and followed him, glorifying God: and all the people, when they saw it, gave praise unto God (Luke 18:43).

Scott knew his brother Dave couldn't have lost weight on his own. Dave had never been able to say no to food in all his life. When he asked Dave who helped him, Dave had just smiled and pointed up into the sky. Scott couldn't believe it. Dave was trying to tell him that God had made the transformation happen? Well, if that was true it would make a believer out of him. Scott had never been much of a Christian before, but if God could do that much for Dave, then He was someone worth believing in. The miracles of God truly are a wonder to behold.

Today's thought: I will glorify God by losing weight for Him and for me!

November 19

Jesus said unto her, I am the resurrection, and the life: he that believeth in me, though he were dead, yet shall he live (John 11:25).

Ralph might as well have been dead. He never went out. He had few friends. He never felt like trying to do anything. He ate and drank and slept and went to work. What a life, if you could call it living. One day he couldn't bring himself to look at his own face in the mirror. Tearfully, he picked up the Bible his dead wife had given him some years before. As he read, he realized how he was throwing his life away. He was somebody important, if for no other reason than that God had made him. With a prayer of thanksgiving on his lips, Ralph decided to make a new start, and God's hand was upon him from that day forward.

Today's thought: I want to live the life God wants me to live!

November 20

Rejoice evermore (1 Thessalonians 5:16).

Fran remembered a time not long ago when she had nothing to smile about. She used to watch other women walk along, and bitter jealousy tore her up inside. She would fly into fits of rage and crying. She hated the way she looked, and she hated other women for looking so good. Her disposition was lousy, and her heart was broken. One Sunday she went to church, and while sitting there, she realized she was at peace. She closed her eyes and prayed, and she felt a voice tell her to change, to do something about her appearance. The impression was so strong that she went home immediately to plan a diet. From that time forward, she never wavered, and now she looked back in amazement. Seventy-five pounds were lost, and joy filled the void they left.

Today's thought: Happiness increases as my weight problem ceases!

November 21

I called upon thy name, O Lord, out of the low dungeon. Thou hast heard my voice: hide not thine ear at my breathing, at my cry (Lamentations 3:55, 56).

The dream was so real. Lew was standing in front of an old house where he could hear a witch cackling in the distance. He knew she was after him, but there was no place to hide. She flew around the corner of the house and touched his arm. At once he began to gain weight. Pound by pound mounted up, until he was a blob of flesh. He couldn't move, and the weight just kept coming. He became a prisoner within a mountainous body. He cried for help, and the clouds parted. A shaft of light came down, and the flesh began to melt. A gentle breeze blew, and Lew knew everything would be all right. When morning came, Lew vowed to lose the pounds he'd unnecessarily put on lately.

Today's thought: From my fleshy prison, I have arisen!

November 22

Praise ye the Lord: for it is good to sing praises unto our God; for it is pleasant; and praise is comely. He healeth the broken in heart, and bindeth up their wounds (Psalms 147:1, 3).

It was more than a diet. For Gary, it was his sanity. He had been obsessed by his weight. He had lived the past three years in a deep and terrible depression. When he was at his lowest, God broke through to him. God turned Gary's life around. He finally began losing weight, and his state of mind improved dramatically. The light of God tore through his darkness with a beautiful healing warmth. Gary was healed of his physical affliction as well as the demon of depression that haunted him. God truly has the power to heal His children. No matter what the problem might be, take it to the Lord.

Today's thought: My diet affects more than just my body; it affects my heart and mind, as well!

November 23

Again, the kingdom of heaven is like unto a merchant man, seeking goodly pearls: who, when he had found one pearl of great price, went and sold all that he had, and bought it (Matthew 13:45, 46).

A diet that worked! It wasn't anything fancy. It wasn't anything expensive. It didn't involve equipment or special treatments. In fact, it was a diet that anyone could do. Sally sat and talked with her pastor for about an hour, and he helped her see why she should diet for her own good, as well as for God. He had been support for her since, and she had included God every step of the way. She felt stronger than ever before. It was like finding a treasure. She was so excited and so thankful. God had given her something that no one else could: a better figure and a deep, abiding joy.

Today's thought: My weight will be lost, no matter the cost!

November 24

When they saw the star, they rejoiced with exceeding great joy (Matthew 2:10).

The star was the sign to the wise men that they were near their journey's end. They had followed the signs of the times, and they had been led toward Bethlehem. The star shone its light on their way, and they came to the Christ child.

As we diet, we can follow the light of Christ in our own lives. Christ shines His light on us to remind us of all we can be. His strength supports us along the way, and we come to possess His joy as we succeed in our quest. Nothing can keep the light of Christ from us, and, with Christ's help, nothing can keep us from losing weight.

Today's thought: If God can lead travelers to the east to find Jesus, then he can lead me to a slimmer, trimmer me!

November 25

And God saw their works, that they turned from their evil way; and God repented of the evil, that he had said that he would do unto them; and he did it not (Jonah 3:10).

Kent was devastated. The police review board had said he would be relieved of active duty if he didn't take off twenty pounds. He was a good cop. How could a few pounds make that much difference? Being a policeman was the most important thing in his life. If losing weight was what was required, then that's what he would do; no two ways about it.

God wants us to do whatever it takes to take care of ourselves. When we do what is right, we escape the bad consequences that come along. Kent knew what he had to do, and he did it. We know what we need to do, and with God's help we, too, will succeed.

Today's thought: It's always a good idea to do what is pleasing to God!

November 26
Then sang Moses and the children of Israel this song unto the Lord, and spake, saying, I will sing unto the Lord for he hath triumphed gloriously: the horse and his rider hath he thrown into the sea (Exodus 15:1).

The children of Israel were pursued by a great army as they came to the Red Sea. The Lord opened their way for them, then closed it up behind them, washing away the fighting force of Egypt. Moses and his followers were delivered, and the power of God was proven once more.

When we are oppressed by obesity, we can also call upon the Savior of Israel for salvation. The God who led His people out of captivity in Egypt will also lead His children of today out of captivity to fat. How can we doubt the power of God? With His help, all things are possible, if we will only believe.

Today's thought: I'm breaking free from a body of fat!

November 27
I say unto you, that likewise joy shall be in heaven over one sinner that repenteth, more than over ninety and nine just persons, which need no repentance (Luke 15:7).

Les dreaded Thanksgiving. He loved his family and friends, and he liked the parades and the football, and he even appreciated the day off from work, but he knew there would be so much tempting food that he wasn't supposed to have. It made him sick to think of all the wonderful things he would have to say no to. He walked up the front sidewalk and rang the bell. He was met by a dozen people who immediately went into raves over how great he looked. He was the topic of conversation the entire day. It wasn't so bad, after all. With everyone complimenting him, he found he had more strength than ever to turn down fattening food.

Today's thought: God will send strength through family and friends!

November 28
And God saw every thing that he had made, and, behold, it was very good. And the evening and the morning were the sixth day (Genesis 1:31).

One thing that makes dieting so hard is that what we have to give up is so good. We have found ways to make foods into so many wonderful concoctions. It would be a lot easier to give up certain foods if they were drab and boring. Yet, variety is a true gift from God. We are given special treats to enjoy, but not to overindulge in. Gluttony robs life of its special treats. When we have whatever we want whenever we want it, then nothing is special anymore. If we will practice discipline and self-restraint, then we can treat ourselves to rich, luscious foods without worry of what they will do to us. That way, we come to enjoy treats the way God meant us to enjoy them.

Today's thought: When I indulge too much, I bulge too much!

November 29
And ye now therefore have sorrow: but I will see you again, and your heart shall rejoice, and your joy no man taketh from you (John 16:22).

It was very weird, but Linda sort of missed her diet. She had made some really good friends in her weight-loss group, and she had gotten used to the routine. If anyone would have told her a few months ago that she would miss dieting, she would have said they were crazy. What was there to miss? She had freedom to eat more of what she wanted to now, and she didn't have to be self-conscious. Linda really believed that God had given her new friends and experiences for a reason. She was so thankful that she had been able to lose weight the way she did, with the people she did. Maybe now she could go back and be a help to others?

Today's thought: On days when I can't help myself, maybe I can help others!

November 30
Let every thing that hath breath praise the Lord. Praise ye the Lord (Psalms 150:6).

The battle wasn't won yet, but Henry felt it was close. He looked better, felt better, and had a more positive attitude. Life was so much more fun, now that he was thinner. All the really hard times were behind him, and he felt his future was pretty bright. God had certainly been good to him. Every day, Henry took time out to thank God for all He had done. Henry didn't know what he'd done to deserve such great blessings, but he wasn't going to question it too much. With God's help, he had been able to do what he could never do before: lose weight!

Today's thought: God's helping me be both lighter of body and lighter of spirit!

DECEMBER
Victory

Christmas is our reminder of the ultimate triumph of Jesus the Christ over life and death. Victory was made available to us all through the tiny babe in Bethlehem. God's power was made our power. The greatest gift of all time was freely given to you and me. As Christian believers, we know our struggles will not be in vain. The Christ who conquered temptation, sickness, and even death gives us the power to be conquerors, also. Christ is the ground of our hope and the promise of our deliverance from the problems that plague us. Though we struggle with our weight, we can rest assured that God will help us lose it, as long as we are faithful and give our best effort. The Lord of all life came to live among us so we might know there is good reason to hold on. The example of our blessed Lord is proof that we can do all things through God, who empowers us. Praise the Lord!

December 1

Nay, in all these things we are more than conquerors through him that loved us (Romans 8:37).

Everyone was impressed with Annette's confidence. One day she announced that she was going on a diet, and she did just that. Over the course of the next few months, people watched the wondrous transformation take place. She had set her mind toward losing weight, and nothing even slowed her down. Such strength of conviction was a great inspiration for her friends.

God loves it when we stand up for something and will not be swayed. Whether it be a matter of faith or just of personal conviction, we are being true to our creator when we triumph. Victory comes to those who walk in confidence.

Today's thought: Without a doubt, fatness is out!

December 2

I press toward the mark for the prize of the high calling of God in Christ Jesus (Philippians 3:14).

When he was young, Luke always came in last. He was never

more than an average student, he had never succeeded much in anything he had done. That all changed when he decided to lose weight. He realized that much of his problem was a lousy self-image. He knew he could succeed, even if no one else did. He would prove it to himself, if nothing else. His pastor had given a sermon called, "Be everything you can be," and Luke was going to give it a shot. God didn't create losers. With God's help, Luke knew he could win. Nothing would stop him now. At long last, Luke was on the road to victory.

Today's thought: I will try to keep my sight on what I want to be soon!

December 3
For whatsoever is born of God overcometh the world: and this is the victory that overcometh the world, even our faith (1 John 5:4).

Sammy was tired of making excuses. He was tired of being dishonest with himself and his friends. He needed to lose weight, and he needed plenty of help to do it. He was considered a strong member of his church, but he didn't even have enough faith or conviction to take off a few pounds. He felt like a hypocrite. Surely, the God who had given him so much strength in other areas of his life could help him lose weight. Christ conquered so very much. Sammy felt he ought to be able to conquer so very little. Prayerfully, he began a journey toward fitness, assured of the victory through his faith in Christ.

Today's thought: A heart full of Christ is more important than a plate full of food!

December 4
Let us draw near with a true heart in full assurance of faith, having our hearts sprinkled from an evil conscience, and our bodies washed with pure water (Hebrews 10:22).

Betty liked having people around. When others watched her, she was more likely to behave herself and stay on her diet. She felt guilty if anyone caught her cheating. A little guilt was a good thing for someone trying to lose weight. When she was alone, she didn't feel nearly as guilty. If she was ever going to lose weight, she was going to have to make sure there were people around.

We ought to remember that no matter what we do, God is watching. He can help us on to victory if we will keep in mind that He is ever with us, to act as our conscience when we need Him to.

Today's thought: I hope my conscience is stronger than my appetite!

December 5

Blessed is the man that endureth temptation: for when he is tried, he shall receive the crown of life, which the Lord hath promised to them that love him (James 1:12).

Shelley was thrilled when she was named homecoming queen. It had been a dream of hers since childhood. When she knew she was in the running, she began to diet. Weight had always been a struggle for her. This time she had great motivation, and that made all the difference in the world. She prayed for God's help, and He gave her the determination she needed to diet — and to win the crown. The crown of the pageant was one thing, but Shelley knew God had given her much more than that. Through faith, she had received life everlasting and a share in the victory of Christ Jesus.

Today's thought: My diet will end, but the lessons learned from it will last a lifetime!

December 6

For thou, Lord, hast made me glad through thy work: I will triumph in the works of thy hands (Psalms 92:4).

Brent never knew how happy he would be when he lost weight. All his life he had toyed with the idea, but the costs always seemed much greater than the benefits. It wasn't until the weight came off that he truly realized how great being thinner really was. He felt better, he looked better, and he enjoyed life in general so much more. He could do things he'd never dreamed of before. Even picking things up off the floor without panting and groaning gave him special pleasure. Brent couldn't thank God enough for helping to find a new life. It was great to be alive!

Today's thought: God makes the joy greater than any amount of sacrifice!

December 7

Then Job answered the Lord, and said, I know that thou canst do every thing, and that no thought can be withholden from thee (Job 42:1, 2).

Blessed assurance. Why do some people seem to have it while others don't? It stems from a very slight difference. Some people know God, and some just believe in Him. Knowing is belief beyond doubt. True confidence in the Lord comes to those who have moved beyond their doubts. When we defeat doubt, then we can enter into a whole new relationship with God and a whole new life. God is greater than any problem we have. If we want to lose weight and want God to help us, we need to know beyond doubt that He will truly help us. Like Job, we need to confess regularly our belief that

147

God can do everything.

Today's thought: If God could create mountains, then He can remove a pound of flesh from me!

December 8

The Lord thy God in the midst of thee is mighty; he will save, he will rejoice over thee with joy; he will rest in his love, he will joy over thee with singing (Zephaniah 3:17).

Toni had a dream that she was entering a room where God was. She couldn't really see Him, but she knew He was there. For some reason, He was very happy with her. He was making her feel very good, and she could tell she had done something to please Him a lot. When she gathered up her nerve, Toni asked God what she had done to make Him so happy. "Lose weight," was the reply. When she awakened, she felt the greatest joy she had ever known. She had really wanted to lose weight for herself, but to think that God was pleased with what she had done made the victory twice as sweet.

Today's thought: I will rejoice with God as the pounds come off!

December 9

And it shall come to pass, that whosoever shall call on the name of the Lord shall be saved (Acts 2:21).

Barbara was so thankful. She had come so far, but lately the stress had been overwhelming. When she was under stress, she liked to eat. She was so afraid of blowing her diet that it just added to the stress. She was nervous and on edge all the time. One evening, while she had some time alone, she settled down to read her Bible and pray. It was one of the most peaceful experiences she had had in weeks. She felt renewed and strengthened by the experience; so much so that she made it a nightly routine. It got her through the stress, and it kept her on her diet. By God's grace, she triumphed.

Today's thought: I admit I need help, but it's good to know that God offers all the help I can handle!

December 10

For the kingdom of God is not meat and drink; but righteousness, and peace, and joy in the Holy Ghost (Romans 14:17).

Joan's doctor had told her to make a list of what was really important to her. Her husband and children headed the list. Her health was next, then her pets. She also wrote down her mother's ring and some furniture that her father had made when he was a young man. Her doctor asked her if she wanted to lose all that was on the list, and she told him, "Of course not!" He told her that she had to lose weight or she wouldn't be around long to enjoy the things she truly loved. If those things were really more important to her than food, then she was going to have to prove it. She asked God for help and then set her mind toward losing weight.

Today's thought: Compared to the truly important things in life, food is pretty pathetic!

December 11

But he that doeth truth cometh to the light, that his deeds may be made manifest, that they are wrought in God (John 3:21).

Jack was so proud to show off his wife, Eileen, when they went home for the holidays. Over the summer and fall, she had lost sixty-five pounds. She looked great, and Jack was proud of her. She had worked so hard, and he felt she deserved some credit. It made Eileen feel good to know it meant so much to Jack. God had been good to them both. He had given them patience to deal with each other, and had blessed them both with strength and encouragement. It was true that when a person worked to do what the Lord wanted her to do, He crowned her in victory and allowed her to bask in the limelight for awhile!

Today's thought: I don't care if I come into the light, as long as I become light!

December 12

Blessed are the pure in heart; for they shall see God (Matthew 5:8).

Denise wanted to do what was right. She was a good person, and it never occurred to her that her weight problem might be displeasing to God. Her friend tried to tell her that it didn't mean God didn't love her. What she meant was that God liked it best when we take the best care of ourselves possible, and that extra weight wasn't doing that. Denise pondered what her friend said to her for a long while, then resolved to try her best to lose weight. Apologetically, she prayed to God and asked Him to help her as she tried to set things right. The prayer of a person pure in heart and full of kindness speaks loudest into the ear of the Lord.

Today's thought: I wish my heart could teach my mouth to say "no!"

December 13

He that hath an ear, let him hear what the Spirit saith unto the churches; To him that overcometh will I give to eat of the tree of life, which is in the midst of the paradise of God (Revelation 2:7).

Beth and David made a deal that they would diet through the week but treat themselves to a night out each week at one of their favorite restaurants. Restaurant night became the best night of the week. Both Beth and David agreed that they had never enjoyed their food so much as when they only splurged one time a week. They grew to appreciate how good it really was. It helped to make even ordinary meals special and delicious.

God has offered us special things to eat. He has created so much to make our lives interesting and varied. We must enjoy these things discreetly and unselfishly. If we will enjoy them within God's plan, then He will reward us with fruit from the tree of life, which will be the finest food we could ever want.

Today's thought: God's food is eternal, and it isn't fattening!

December 14

For ye have need of patience, that, after ye have done the will of God, ye might receive the promise (Hebrews 10:36).

Paula woke up in pain. Her stomach was cramping, and she felt ill. It must have been the diet pills. Her friend had told her they were safe and they'd help her take off weight three times as fast as normal. Why had she listened to her? She knew pills weren't the answer, but she wanted to lose weight fast. She never had been very good on patience. Her mother told her to pray for patience, but no, Paula thought she had a better idea. The truth was, there was only one way she was going to lose weight, and that was through perseverance and patience. Her mother was right. If God would give her a second chance, maybe together they could make it work.

Today's thought: Nothing takes off weight faster than devotion and commitment!

December 15

For he that is mighty hath done to me great things; and holy is his name (Luke 1:49).

Carolyn felt good about herself. She was in her own apartment, working full time at a job she loved, and she was looking better than ever before. God had been so good to her. She was afraid when she first set out on her own, but she knew He was looking after her. With God on her side, she felt she could accomplish anything. God had set her feet on a good road, and she was going to try her hardest to stick to it. She wanted everyone to know what God had done for her, and she planned to do nothing that would allow anyone to doubt. The power of God shone brightly through her life, and she was glad.

Today's thought: I want my diet to be a sign of God's grace!

December 16
Blessed be the Lord, who daily loadeth us with benefits, even the God of our salvation. Selah (Psalms 68:19).

Doris stood at the window, watching the first heavy snow cover everything outside with a blanket of white. She sipped a cup of tea and reflected on the year quickly fleeting. So many good things had happened. Certainly there had been bad, too, but mostly it was good. She couldn't imagine why she was so lucky as to have so many things going her way. The Lord had looked kindly on her this year. She had never felt so healthy and good. The year had seen weight loss every month. She finally was beginning to look like she'd always dreamed she could. The Lord could take credit for that, too. There was no way Doris could have done so well if God hadn't strengthened her.

Today's thought: I gladly receive all the benefits the Lord has to give, as long as they're not fattening!

December 17
Know ye not that they which run in a race run all, but one receiveth the prize? So run, that ye may obtain (1 Corinthians 9:24).

Todd wasn't getting anywhere with his diet. It was on and off, at best. He just couldn't stick to it. He'd never been good at discipline and conditioning. How many times had he been kicked off high school teams for not practicing? He just didn't have the killer instinct. He didn't want to win badly enough.

We'll have difficulty losing weight if our heart isn't really in it. If we're going to run the race for weight loss, then we need to be serious about winning it. Pray that God will strengthen both your heart and body, so that when the race is finished, you receive the prize.

Today's thought: Help me remember that I'm not just running away from fat, but that I'm running toward God's design of who I should be!

December 18
For where your treasure is, there will your heart be also (Matthew 6:21).

Grady thought he was pretty smart, hiding the chocolate bars beside his bed. He would do well on his diet during the day, but at night he would go wild eating chocolate. Every day he would talk a good game, saying how much he really wanted to be thinner, but when the lights went out at night, he would undo all his fine talk by sneaky, fattening action. When he was caught, Grady merely shrugged it off, saying he wouldn't do it again. The next night, Grady fell asleep with chocolate thick on his breath. Actions often do speak louder than words. Where our treasure is — that is, what's really important to us — there will our hearts and actions be, also.

Today's thought: Make my diet important enough to me to keep me from temptation!

December 19

Now no chastening for the present seemeth to be joyous, but grievous: nevertheless afterward it yieldeth the peaceable fruit of righteousness unto them which are exercised thereby (Hebrews 12:11).

Jeremy was good for her. Whenever she did something she shouldn't or ate something that wasn't on her diet, he was quick to chastise her for it. She hated when he did it, but that made it all the more effective. There were times she wanted to throttle him, but most of the time she wanted to kiss him. He was the reason her dieting was working, and though sometimes it was annoying, she wouldn't change it for anything.

God will help keep us in line, if we let Him. We need someone to watch over us; to keep us out of mischief. God will make sure we last until we triumph, if we will allow Him to do so.

Today's thought: The call of fattening food is not as loud as the call of God to do what's right!

December 20

To him that overcometh will I grant to sit with me in my throne, even as I also overcame, and am set down with my Father in his throne (Revelation 3:21).

Gramps promised Kathy that if she would lose forty pounds by Christmas, he would take her to Bermuda with him. Kathy could hardly wait for Gramps to see her. She'd topped out at fifty-three pounds lost, and had a note from her doctor as documented proof. At first, she never thought she'd make it, but a lot of prayers, sweat, tears, and sacrifice had made it come true. She had never worked so hard for anying in her life. Even without the trip, she felt she'd received reward enough, but she planned to hold Gramps to his promise, anyway.

Today's thought: I'd rather be overjoyed than overweight!

December 21

Now thanks be unto God, which always causeth us to triumph in Christ, and maketh manifest the savour of his knowledge by us in every place (2 Corinthians 2:14).

Rose was hoping for some miracle to appear in her Christmas stocking. Another year was almost gone, and she hadn't lost any weight. Each year she swore things would be different, and nothing ever changed. Rose just didn't have any commitment at all. She knew no one would lose the weight for her, but she kept hoping it would melt away on its own.

Dreaming won't make our weight disappear. We need to take positive steps on our own. However, we have God to help us. He will carry us when we are too weak to continue, and He will encourage us when we feel depressed and hopeless. God offers us victory in the face of failure. Accept God's help, and a miracle will indeed happen.

Today's thought: I know what I need to do to lose weight, and with God's help I will do it!

December 22

Brethren, I count not myself to have apprehended: but this one thing I do, forgetting those things which are behind, and reaching forth unto those things which are before (Philippians 3:13).

Wendy had a hard time putting her past behind her. Christmas had been torture for her as a child. Everyone would talk about "poor" Wendy, who was fat and awkward. Everyone always picked on her, and they never let her eat the things she wanted. Every single person had some sage bit of advice for her. Even though things had changed a lot in the past couple of years, she still dreaded the holidays. She was trim and svelte, and no one could do anything but admire her, and still it was hard. Old demons die hard.

Dieting requires much more than physical transformation. It also calls for emotional healing, and the one sure source for that is God.

Today's thought: The past is fast fading away. I'm headed for a trimmer me!

December 23

Who hath delivered us from the power of darkness, and hath translated us into the kingdom of his dear Son (Colossians 1:13).

Christmas was going to be extra fun this year. Lois hadn't told anyone that she had lost a good deal of weight. More than that, she had been so depressed by her weight problem in the past that she hadn't been much fun to be around. She felt so much better about herself, and she definitely felt better about the holidays. Her life had been lived in the darkness of depression, but the light of God had broken through, much like the star of Bethlehem broke through the Jerusalem sky two thousand years before. The wise men had found the baby Jesus by following its light, and Lois had found a new life of her own, led by the very same saving light of God.

Today's thought: The lightness of my body is due to the light of Christ!

December 24

And the Lord direct your hearts into the love of God, and into the patient waiting for Christ (2 Thessalonians 3:5).

Nancy sat in the warm glow of the firelight, looking at the sparkle of the Christmas tree. What was it like that very first Christmas morn? What must Mary and Joseph have been feeling? Imagine the anticipation and wonder. Nancy's mind wandered to the fact that she had lost so much weight through the year. Suddenly, she was embarrassed by a thought. She had thought her diet was so important, she had been so impatient trying to lose weight. Compared with the magic and wonder of this night, and all that it meant, her diet seemed pretty insignificant. She owed everything she had and everything she was to Jesus Christ. It was a joy to welcome Him into her heart once again this blessed Christmas Eve.

Today's thought: The day-to-day gifts of God pale in comparison with His greatest gift: His Son, Jesus the Christ!

December 25

Herein is love, not that we loved God, but that he loved us, and sent his Son to be the propitiation for our sins (1 John 4:10).

God has given all to make us happy. He has blessed us with a beautiful world, a wonderful life, and many opportunities for fulfillment and joy. He asks that we respect His gifts and endeavor to be the best people we can possibly be. To help us, He sent His only Son to come into this world as an example. We can know God's desire for us through His Son. Not only did His Son come as an example, but as a Savior, to allow us to be reconciled with our God. All that we have received is from God. On this glorious Christmas morn, make a gift of your life to God. Give Him the only thing that truly matters: *You.*

Today's thought: If I can in any way be used, help me bring about peace on earth and goodwill to all God's children!

December 26

For our light affliction, which is but for a moment, worketh for us a far more exceeding and eternal weight of glory (2 Corinthians 4:17).

The army had been good for Stan. When he was younger, he was completely undisciplined. The army had taken care of that. He had to work his tail off to get into good shape, but it was worth it. The short period of affliction he suffered through helped him in so many other ways. The folks back home couldn't believe the change they saw while he was home for the holidays.

God disciplines His children on occasion because He knows the lasting lessons we need to learn. Diets help us do a lot more than just lose weight. Diets discipline us and help us grow in maturity and fitness for the kingdom of God.

Today's thought: A gain in discipline means a loss in weight!

December 27

He that hath an ear, let him hear what the Spirit saith unto the churches; To him that overcometh will I give to eat of the hidden manna, and will give him a white stone, and in the stone a new name written, which no man knoweth saving he that receiveth it (Revelation 2:17).

Donna thanked God for giving her a whole new life. Losing the weight had only been part of it. Donna had fervently prayed for transformation, but she never bargained for all that God would do for her. Her attitude was transformed from one of doom to one of hope. Her appearance was transformed from one of dumpiness to one of beauty. Her emotional stability had been transformed from one of teetering on the brink to solid rock. She couldn't believe it, but she was a totally different person than she had been a year before. The God of miracles and life had certainly worked in Donna's life. He's available to work in ours, also.

Today's thought: With God's help I will lose weight, lose hate, and lose my desire to denigrate!

December 28

Who is he that overcometh the world, but he that believeth that Jesus is the Son of God? (1 John 5:5.)

Burt couldn't help but rub it in. Terry had claimed to have found the diet breakthrough of the century. He lost seven pounds. Greg got hold of some miracle pills, and he lost eleven pounds. Craig had mortgaged his house to buy a membership in a health club. He managed to lose fourteen pounds. Burt had simply told his friends he was going to lose weight on the Jesus plan. Whenever he got hungry between meals, he was going to go off and read the gospels. They had all laughed long and hard at him, but he who laughs last, laughs best. Twenty-eight pounds had dropped from the Jesus plan. There's nothing like it.

Today's thought: God can do for me what nothing on earth can!

December 29

Then the devil leaveth him, and, behold, angels came and ministered unto him (Matthew 4:11).

Victory! Steve felt he'd really run the good race. No matter how great the temptations had gotten lately, he had been able to withstand them. Christ was pulling him through the roughest times yet. Each time he beat back the temptations, he felt better than ever. It was as if God was rewarding him by making him feel so good. The pounds were coming off, and it was actually beginning to get easy. Steve never thought he'd come to say that. Steve was convinced. If God could make a diet tolerable, then God really could do anything!

Today's thought: I will not take part in devil's food!

December 30

Whether therefore ye eat, or drink, or whatsover ye do, do all to the glory of God (1 Corinthians 10:31).

Leah remembered the question her pastor had asked, "What do you think God wants you to eat?" At first, it had seemed like a silly question, but the more Leah thought about it, the more she realized there really wasn't any food God didn't want to let her have. It was the quantities and frequency of consumption that Leah realized God would disapprove of. Moderation in everything was the rule she needed to follow. She felt so much better. Her diet didn't need to be a lot of heavy sacrifices. All she needed to do was develop some self-control, and with God's help, she would.

Today's thought: Let my eating and drinking offend no one, especially God!

December 31

Go thy way, eat thy bread with joy, and drink thy wine with a merry heart; for God now accepteth thy works (Ecclesiastes 9:7).

There will come a day when the diet is truly over. We must endure until that day with a strong spirit and an earnest desire to please the Lord. We have been blessed with much, and in some cases, too much. God has been good to give, and He will be equally good to help take away. Remember the Lord every step of your diet. Call upon Him for strength, for comfort, for hope, and for courage. He will hear you, and He will be sure to answer you. In time, you will come to that day, not too distant, when you can eat your bread with joy and without guilt, drink and make merry, and stand confident and proud that you have indeed glorified your Lord.

Today's thought: I will be a conqueror, through the mighty love of God.

May the peace of God abide with you always, the love of Christ protect you from the storms of life, and the power of the Holy Spirit strengthen you all the days of your life. Amen.